A QUANTUM HEALING EX^{2}PRESSION

*An Intelligent **Living** Information Field Expression*

By

Dr. George A. Munger PhD

PUBLISHING INFORMATION

FIRST EDITION

Library of Congress Registration Number: TXu 2178-076 (Copyright 2019)

ISBN: 978-0-578-22969-0

WGAWEST REGISTRY No. 2028342

ISBN 978-0-578-22969-0

9 780578 229690 >

DISCLAIMER

It is never my intention to provide specific medical advice to readers, but rather to provide information to help them better understand their health, previously diagnosed conditions, self-healing awareness and the various options related to treatment of disease, prevention, supportive care and nutrition. The reader accepts all responsibility to contact their doctor(s) and is strongly advised to contact other licensed health professionals from around the world to receive the most current information which is pertinent to their specific medical condition. Consult with a doctor of your choice or, better yet, all of the following: Your personal doctor, Nutritionist, Acupuncturist, Homeopathic practitioner, Pharmacist, Naturopathic practitioner, Ayurvedic doctor, Tibetan doctor, Integrative medicine doctor, Oncologist and patients whom are survivors of the same disease or malady you have been diagnosed with. Then, using all this information, make your decision based on what you believe to be reasonable and reliable.

Neither this book nor the author is responsible for the quality of the information or services provided by other organizations mentioned on websites, nor do we endorse any services, product, treatment, or therapy.

Disclaimers, like the one you are reading, are utilized to mitigate or eliminate liability regarding the information contained in this book. We ask that you use common sense. More information is better than less. Please consult with a licensed doctor or medical professional when evaluating any type of medical modality or treatment referenced within the pages of this book or presented to you in any other manner.

Invincible ignorance has become a Reality Replication Template which has penetrated all areas of reason. This un-awareness creates systems of interference in our scientific quest for information. Choose wisely when referencing medical modalities and treatments. Always ask questions of your doctor(s). Have faith, for the truth will withstand all scrutiny.

DEDICATION

A resounding thank you is sincerely expressed to my son Michael and to all the innovative thinkers in search of scientific and spiritual truth. It is my hope the small observations and discoveries noted in this book inspire greater contributions. I thank all seekers for pushing the boundaries of knowledge and embracing the global illumination caused by sowing the seeds of scientific change. Thank you for casting off the burdens inherent in diploma mill indoctrination, systems of interference, professional ostracism and all other forms of prejudice that skews data or confers bias. Thank you for your professional integrity which applauds the personal responsibility of all who formulate new ideas which incorporate un-biased data into their research and rejects data which predisposes compliance with pre-existing conclusions or systems of interference. Thank you for your individual steadfast participation in the search for a truth which embraces change and logically presents the research community and the planet with an example to be duplicated. My passion, my inspiration and my compass are by-products of your examples. You are instrumental toward awakening me, the scientific community, and the rest of humanity. Thank you!

ACKNOWLEDGEMENTS

I wish to gratefully acknowledge ALL those whose help and insights have increased the readability of this book.

Michael J. Munger

Dr. Michelle Halvorson

Marilyn O'Day

Linda Jo Safford

Briana Newcomer

Lara Greenberg

Dennis Burke

Ricky Keeler

Grey Nagele

Cindy Draughon

Paul Howe

TABLE OF CONTENTS

Preface

Many types of knowledge and perception exist in secret compartments hidden from us in our *un-awareness*. This un-awareness is perceived in your mind as a state of "not knowing". However, this is not just your un-awareness, it is an un-awareness experienced by us as a species. Through the process of discovery (intentional and unintentional), we uncover these secret compartments. All discoveries are interpreted with our pre-existing knowledge and perceptions. However, predicated on these discoveries is a fact which insists some discoveries have the potential to change the course of human thought. This book is about these quantum leaps of awareness.

Humanity has been writing, researching, and hypothesizing about its own existence since before the beginning of recorded thought. The discoveries elucidated in this book have evolved due to the combined thoughts of *all* humans and all organisms imbued with intelligent live information field expressions, LIFE (explained later). Without acknowledging the input from the rest of the human continuum, these discoveries would not have been possible. It would indeed be arrogant to claim these discoveries as my own—they are ours. It is my sincere hope that others, with their individual specific perceptions, will discover the awareness expressions I have encountered and utilize them to illuminate themselves and evolve our species.

My name is Dr. George A. Munger PhD, I am an Asian medicine practitioner with an emphasis on self-healing, preventative medicine, integrative medicine and living plant medicine (Arizona license #0776). My observations offer a new perspective of existing knowledge and opens the door to new concepts about life. Many new equations and concepts are used in this book. These were created and introduced by me. They are based on my experience with patients and my dissertation regarding Quantum Phyto-Sapience (quantum plant intelligence; an information field) which I submitted to satisfy part of the requirements for my Doctorate and PhD in Quantum Medicine. These new discoveries are based on logical extrapolations of data gleaned from multiple published studies, some of which I piggy-backed my own research onto (these have been cited and gratefully acknowledged). This endeavor required years of work to extrapolate and has demanded diligent logic to prove—an enlightenment which has turned into an on-going discovery of self-healing, plant-healing, self-awareness, and information expressions.

It does not matter what type of imbalance or disease you are experiencing, there are examples of documented medical phenomenon, actual case histories of self-healing, which have resulted in a cure or remission of that disease or malady. These examples travel beyond the current understanding of medical science and include miracle cures, spontaneous remissions, and placebo effects. These are examples of self-healing or life-directed healing. You will learn that your specific degree of self-healing awareness greatly enhances, supports, and augments any medical treatment protocol. These phenomena are also documented as in-explicable stand-alone cures. If you are searching to find out who you are and what makes you tick, *A Quantum Healing Ex²pression* will provide a new and unique perspective, which will change you forever!

This book addresses the difference between "curing" and "healing". You will be taught how to create an individual specific template that allows you to take control of your life and enhance your self-healing through the creation of an individual specific Reality Replication Template (explained later).

The logical and innovative approaches to healing introduced in this book will strengthen all aspects of your life; not just address dis-ease. You have an opportunity to connect to a new way of living that is replicateable and sustainable. Together, we will un-cover *your* path. A path which will lead to awareness, self-awareness, self-healing, and positive change. This is my gift to you and our gift to the rest of humanity.

Introduction

"Life as a whole expresses itself as a force that is not to be contained within any one part." –Goethe

"All healing is self-healing predicated on your perception of this awareness."—Dr. G. Munger

"Essentially, your environment, your intention or both, can modify your existing genome."—Dr. G. Munger

It is time to set sail for the quantum adventure of a life-time—for you are embarking on a voyage of discovery. Together, we will uncover the forgotten knowledge of humans and experience new knowledge which will dramatically improve your life, career, relationships, health, and finances, and allow you to find your true self. By reading this book, you are sailing in the flow of time, experiencing a new awareness— "now is the only time change ever happens. This secret knowledge is predicated on discovery, and discovery is predicated on awareness. Let us begin…

There was no doubt about it; I was just like any other student in a PhD program—totally immersed in writing my dissertation and stressed to the max. I kept focus on my goal—a goal which would eventually allow me to receive my Doctorate and PhD in Quantum Medicine.

There I was, close to finishing my dissertation for the *fourth* time! It seemed like every time I neared the end of my research, I observed something else that needed to be included and *proven.* Work, work, work; it seemed endless.

On this occasion, I was plagued with how plants collect, and record information gleaned from their environment (plant awareness). I could observe it, but I could not prove it—yet). I was at the end of my rope, exhausted, burnt out and brain dead. I pondered whether I would ever be able to prove how an intelligent plant collects data (insert cuss word here). All I knew was the current definition of "plant intelligence" was incomplete, antiquated, anthropomorphic and not useable. For all intents and purposes, it was non-existent. All I was doing was getting more frustrated.

I decided to take a break and visit my favorite coffee shop just to do some people watching and veg-out. I ordered a chai tea latte, my favorite, and a pastry. I should have done this sooner. Sipping my tea quickly relaxed me and before I knew it, I was whispering, "Umm, this tastes good" and dropping pastry crumbs all over myself and the table. I was looking a group of students sitting at a table near the front window. They were laughing and having fun. Ahh! those were the days. Then, right in the middle of taking another sip of tea, it hit me. Seemingly out of nowhere, a sudden awareness of "knowing" occurred. I quickly grabbed my pen and began to write down this new knowledge -- a knowledge that would change my life forever.

This new knowledge made me aware that humans were collecting and recording their life experiences in a manner that was completely different from what I was taught in school (diploma mill indoctrination). But, more importantly, I realized I had just received this knowledge as if by magic. It just popped into my mind. Where did this come from? I knew it could not have come from my brain because I had not experienced this thought or insight of knowledge until now. What I mean by this is it was not recorded in my brain until ***after*** I experienced the "knowing" in my mind. So, where did this new knowledge come from?

I was excited and in awe. This was incredible! Unfortunately, there was nothing tangible I could latch on to. There just was not anything there; literally. You cannot get something from nothing. Yet here it was. What was I missing? Was I tired?

I have read about "instantaneous knowing" in the past—I experienced it a year ago. This latest insight was identical to what I experienced then. However, when this happened to me the previous time, I was so excited with the information I received that I gave little thought to how it occurred. I took my gift of new knowledge and applied it to whatever I was analyzing at the time and moved on.

But this time was different! This sudden awareness of knowledge provided *a process of how this access occurs*—one of the reasons for writing this book.

A new awareness template was forming in my mind which allowed me to receive information from some unknown place. I experienced a nagging sense this "sudden knowing" must have a physical location, yet it presented itself as intangible and invisible (Yeah, I know). Nevertheless, I was intrigued and drawn forward. The more I tried to locate where this information came from, the more I was able to receive additional information. As if the enigma that is me was not perplexing enough, I was now contemplating how *all information* is transmitted and recorded by all humans. I was excited beyond imagination. Then I slumped over for a second and sighed, "This new "knowing" is about humans and not about plants—I will never finish my dissertation." Nevertheless, my mind kept racing and analyzing until I realized I was wrong! It was not just about humans; it impacted *all* life forms.

To say this was a little overwhelming is an understatement. How can you define a process which is *individually specific* to the tune of 7.7 billion interpretations not including other life forms, in a manner that helps others experience the same "access" I experienced? I reasoned that if I was experiencing this, then I might be able to utilize the same source which created the "knowing awareness" for me in the first place. These were uncharted waters; I dove in.

Five minutes ago, I had been so tired, exhausted, and burned out that I forced myself to take a break. Now I was so pre-occupied with this new knowledge that I could not sleep (welcome to research). My head was spinning with possibilities. I could not stop thinking this must be a "field" comprised of individual thought images or pictures which somehow interfaced with my mind (tell me that does not sound nutso). As most of you have guessed, this field is not the kind of field where crops are grown. It is a field that can be likened to an electro-magnetic field, a gravitational field, or other force field. A field comprised of thought images (information) or *expressions of light*—pictures. Additionally, I could record these "thought expressions" of pictures in my brain should I want to. I realized I was receiving holographic images, or pictures, and *not* text or raw environmental sensory data. More importantly, it was going directly into my mind and *by-passing my senses* which all of us normally use to collect information. To add to the complexity of this experience, these images were immediately interpreted and translated into my native tongue—in this case English (What?). This made it even more intriguing. Are photonic images which are embedded or encoded with information a universal language? I kept asking myself question after question. This "knowing" created an awareness in me of a "field" which accumulates thought images; images which I could access. More importantly, these images were embedded with information which I could decipher and understand. Ah! Have I discovered an information field which I never knew existed until now? If these data are presented as pictures, I reasoned, then they must be *frequencies of light*—a frequency of the electromagnetic spectrum of radiation. After all, it was a holographic image or picture; right? I wanted to get this straight. My mind was somehow able to receive images of visible frequencies of light from a field which stored light images! Additionally, these images had information embedded into them which I could decipher using my own language. These images were perceived by me to be intelligent, organized and easily understood. How did this "knowledge" make instantaneous sense to me? (Dang! More questions.) I immediately sensed this was important and should be shared with everyone. As you will see, this was just the tip of the iceberg, so to speak.

However, I quickly found out explaining it to others would prove challenging. I mean, how could I instantaneously understand something so complex, yet be required to coin new words to explain my observations to others? (I guess "a picture is worth a thousand words"—Fred R. Barnard, a variation of his original quote). Furthermore, the data which presented itself to me created an "awareness" in my mind which gave me the *option* to record it in my brain. In other words, it was not forced upon me—I had a choice. I could take it or leave it (it was fortunate I had a crumb and tea-soaked napkin to write this stuff down on).

I kept thinking this field could only be accomplished by something that was intelligent and organized… Then, bam! Another flash of instantaneous knowing hit me. I realized the field that stored this information was intelligent, organized, and *alive.* Oh no! Here come the men in white coats. Hey, what was in that tea? Was I out of touch with reality? Or finally getting in touch with reality? How could a field of photonic images be intelligent and alive? I have never heard of such a thing. Nevertheless, if my mind could receive these images and my brain could record these images, then it is possible to directly experience information images that carry data *not* generated in my physical environment or my brain. As you will see, proving this information field is alive and intelligent is a logical extrapolation. Everything was changing.

In this book we will discuss and analyze how this happens. You will personally experience an important aspect of this information. An aspect which states the memories in your brain are *pictures, or images* which are associated with sensory data and the carriers of this information, Photon Information Expressions (PIEs) radiating from an information field. This process culminates in your mind as images. These images transmit and record data into your brain. In other words, an "information image" is transmitted to your mind on a photonic frequency of the electromagnetic spectrum of radiation, and then your mind records this information in your brain as an information encoded image (this will be explained completely in Chapter 5, Photonic Encoding). I believe this is observed as one of the unknown aspects of the process known as neurogenesis. Neurogenesis is a process that creates a physical manifestation of a neuron to store information in the brain. Now, it appears the information storing process is photon-related which imprints data (encodes) on a picture, *not the actual sensory data*. In other words, your invisible and non-material mind tells your physical brain to create a place to store this information. This is "intended" by you and stored in your brain in the form of a picture! This discovery creates a new perspective which utilizes "thought expressions" as photon information carriers. It provides a new way of how information is perceived and interpreted by your mind and then recorded in your brain. As if this is not extraordinary enough, I came to learn these pictures are not only experienced in your mind and stored in your brain, but are transmitted and stored in what I call a Total Information Continuum (TIC) which is part of a quantum "information field". I call this an intelligent Live Information Field Expression (LIFE). This is the physical place I sensed my "instantaneous knowing" came from. Do not worry, you will quickly understand this new knowledge, as it will be broken down into small bits of information, so it is easy to understand. This book will employ a logical extrapolation and analysis of these scientific observations (quantum thought expressions) creating a bridge which connects scientific method and spiritual analysis. Please remember, science and spiritual interpretations are inseparable—two forms of information awareness blurred by semantics, prejudice, and thousands of years of rigid doctrine.

As I fell down my quantum rabbit hole, my awareness experiences kept changing until they reached a point where they created a new perspective of my current knowledge and consequently, my awareness. This is the awareness perspective I hope you will choose to embrace. You will undoubtedly experience access to a Living Intelligent Field using a thought expression, but *only* if you intend this to happen. Please remember "choice" creates everything (even not choosing is a choice). This book will show you how to master this and create a permanent change in your awareness—a change which makes you self-aware. I know this sounds crazy, but sometimes there is no way of stating an observation except to just come out and say it. Are the guys in the white coats gone? Good, let us continue.

Initially, the researchers I shared this with wanted to take me to a veterinarian and have me put down. (Ha! friends, you got to love 'um.) If you do not know this already, humans resist new awareness which does not seamlessly integrate with their current mind set or what I call their Reality Replication Template, their repeated egoic sense of self. However, once these folks got past their preference for comfortable and familiar knowledge, they quickly came around and were intrigued by the possibilities of this discovery. Nevertheless, these discoveries will undoubtedly affect *your* knowledge, *your* perception, and create a new awareness in you. Come with me and learn to see the world in a unique way—an enlightened way (pun intended).

If we peek inside and ask, "How long has this quantum field of intelligent information been around?" you will see that this type of eternal knowledge *insists* on being recorded as pictures (photonic expressions) and is consequently part of our eternal quantum cyclic existence. As you will learn, information appears to exist forever. Once recorded, it is forever imbedded in photonic expressions (otherwise, you could not discover it. You would have to invent it). You will learn awareness is required to detect these discoveries. This observation is how all information is updated in the human awareness experience, and includes the information required to create self-awareness and is related to the focus of this book. Awareness is a thought expression and part of LIFE.

All healing is self-healing. Regardless of the medical modality used to help cure an ailment, in the end, it is the *patient* that heals herself or himself. Your choice of healing modality either facilitates or inhibits this process. Additionally, your *level* of self-healing awareness also facilitates or inhibits this process. Remember, *all* humans have varying degrees of self-healing and self-awareness.

You will discover varying degrees of self-healing are possible even *without* your knowing about it—you do it every day. Self-healing exhibits an intelligent Live Information Field Expression that radiates Photonic Information Expressions (PIEs are explained later) which are received by your physical body. The efficacy of the healing response is dependent on the physical body's ability to utilize these PIE emissions (observed as your state of health) and is strongly mitigated by your awareness of this healing response. As mentioned above, this happens to some degree regardless of your current level of awareness. However, self-healing can be *increased dramatically* with the realization and utilization of self-awareness. In this book, awareness is predicated on one's choice to utilize or discard an intended "thought expression" with the goal being fulfillment of a healing "intention". For our purposes in this book, self-awareness is defined as detection, or the ability to be cognizant, of a thought that is happening to you both physically and mentally as well as how you express your quantum self. Any awareness creates change, either positive or negative, and it is chosen by you. If you choose to ignore self-awareness you will continue to create your life the same way you have always experienced it, unaware of your quantum gift—the ability to create change.

However, you would not be reading this book if that were the case. We search because we believe in quantum possibilities. You will learn how to embrace and utilize self-awareness and, in the process, discover a new understanding of the individual specific person known as *you*. By utilizing “intent”, this understanding is unavoidable. Once you know, you cannot un-know. However, you can replace this knowing with new knowing—a quantum leap. *A Quantum Healing Ex²pression* provides insights that allow you to create and orchestrate a more functional understanding of this complex quantum process.

A live field (a LIFE force) emanates from your living body as is does from all living things. The feeling of being alive comes from your recognition of this field emanation. You will learn you do not die! Instead you experience a death-transition. This transition is the separation of the physical body from your *observation* of an animated “live field, force or power” emanating from your living body (or any living body). This is an intelligent Live Information Field Expression or force you recognize as being alive. The life force or power is an intelligent field expression that cannot be destroyed (it is not material). You will learn a living intelligent field of information is present, in varying degrees, in ***all*** living organisms. Additionally, this information field works in conjunction with ***all*** medical modalities and treatment protocols, even if you impede this process by being unaware.

You will discover a new awareness of your environment. This new awareness will help you understand how data intrusion from your environment and your thought expressions can alter your genome, or genetic makeup. **Essentially, your environment, your intention or *both*, can modify your existing genome.** Your DNA (blueprint) is just part of this equation. DNA is a plan for building a living organism, it is *not the builder*.

This book will expand on the medical research of tens of thousands of complex self-healings that defied the odds of this statistical norm. You will find there are more proven examples of spontaneous remission, miracle cures and placebo effect than what was previously thought. However, we will not cover the billions and billions of common self-healings that occur daily, because they are self-evident. For instance, sneezing, coughing, vomiting, tearing, nasal mucous discharge, scratching, swelling, fever, blisters, pain, sleep, the inflammation response, or scabs forming over a scrape in order to protect and regenerate damaged tissue—the list goes on. Instead, we will investigate examples of self-healing that are much more complex—the placebo effect, spontaneous remission of cancer, and miracle-cure experiences. These examples are observed as the result of self-healing. A healing which utilizes "information" transmitted from LIFE, via PIEs to *your* mind and then to your physical body with instructions which facilitate a specific healing equation (it appears everyone can recall having experienced self-healing. You just needed someone to point it out to you again). Additionally, if you have not observed your body as a compounding pharmacy, you should consider this observation.

How can we, as humans, support and augment our awareness of this innate healing information process? One of the goals of this book is to answer these questions and to provide a template to guide you through your own individual healing awareness development. Your perception of yourself will be changed after reading this book—the change is inevitable. This book demonstrates that healing awareness is not only exhibited by the physical body, it also occurs in the mind and the quantum or spiritual aspects of your existence as well. You will see that emotions (love, hate, fear and many others) have a profound effect on your health (*Emotions are thought expressions originating in the mind and experienced in both the mind and body. A mind/body connection exists in all humans*.

Science and spirit are not as far apart as one might have heard. Scientific awareness and self-awareness support the consciousness related to knowledge, perception, and self-healing. This book explains how scientific awareness, spiritual awareness and consciousness are integrated into the shared reality we call life on earth. It offers an opportunity to expand your knowledge of scientific awareness which creates a bridge to a spiritual consciousness (a quantum concept). I believe spiritual consciousness is a quantum field expression or a God expression. Please remember, science and spirit co-exist and are inseparable. You will be given the opportunity to evolve your understanding of your awareness. Choosing to know will undoubtedly create profound healing effects in your life that are dependent on your specific awareness and the way *you choose* to use it. Get ready to remove your mask of social conformity and reveal the real you—a process that will show you how you became you.

Chapter 1

"Scientific evidence of any kind should never be omitted—systems of interference of any kind should never be included."
—Dr. G. Munger

How You Create You

Before you start reading this chapter, I ask that you indulge me by making an awareness observation of yourself—think about how you became the person you are today. There is no right or wrong answer, but the observation will pre-dispose you to receive the following information. *A Quantum Healing Ex²pression* will teach you how "you" came to exist and how you continue to create your individual specific existence. Furthermore, we will provide direction on how to use your "intention", a quantum expression, to create change. OK, here we go!

First, we must establish a premise of how "we" create our physical bodies, our mental awareness—our interpretation of our lives. Additionally, we need to describe some of the ways we collect data to support these assertions. To accomplish this, we will develop an elementary understanding of how you become you. This understanding will be presented in a straightforward step by step format to insure ease of use and replication. We will discuss and analyze human senses and how they play a crucial role in your individual self-development. Along with this, we will discuss ways to glean information using different approaches for gathering data, like using the Lock-on Lock-out principle and two new definitions coined by me to prevent the confusion inherent in the existence of multiple definitions used to describe bias, skewed data and ego based observations. I call these Systems of Interference and Reality Replication Templates.

Let us start with a typical way to collect information which provides us with an example of how to count, measure, and understand physical presentations of data known as quantitative methodology. You have done this type of information collection many times during your life's journey.

Quantitative Methodology

University of Southern California defines quantitative methodology as "Methods which emphasize objective measurements and the statistical, mathematical or numerical analysis of data collected through polls, questionnaires, and surveys, or by manipulating pre-existing statistical data using computational techniques. Quantitative research focuses on gathering numerical data and generalizing it across groups of people or to explain a particular phenomenon." [1]

This type of scientific research approach collects information in a very logical manner. If we allow the following to represent a simple example for collecting observed science data (empirical observations), it will include material representations, statistics, mathematics, or data compiled using direct examination of case studies or real time examples. After measuring the data, one needs to replicate the results. Preferably, this would be completed by having other researchers in the same field of study examine the same problem and utilize the same methods of investigation. If the results match, then voila! Proof of concept or hypothesis is provided—there is an agreement.

The above-mentioned definition can be expressed like this: Definition of the problem + quantification of data + replication of results = proof of concept or proof of hypothesis or **(D+Q+ROR = Proof)**. However, and *this is a big however*, empirical science also provides a definition [2] as follows: Definition of the problem + replication of results = proof of concept or **(D + ROR = Proof)**. The measuring of the data has been left out! This definition is used when material measurement is not possible, and when non-material data is observed *as present*, but not quantifiable. In these instances, the non-material observations need to be included in the analysis, otherwise this would be an example of Systems of Interference, SI. All we need to do is use a separate method, an approach known as qualitative methodology, to account for these non-material observations. Do not let this throw you off course. This is just accounting for the observations that are not material and cannot be measured physically. Nevertheless, we need to include this invisible and non-material information because it can be logically concluded to exist. The replication or end-result is *exhibited as a material form*. This is super-important!

For example: Spontaneous remission of cancer has been documented by Dr. Kelly A. Turner, Ph.D., author of "Radical Remission: Surviving Cancer against All Odds" [3] et.al. However, science has not been able to explain how or why this occurs.

In this case, the replicated spontaneous remission results are observable and exhibit as a verifiable material construct—you can see it. It is the process of *how* this happens, that is unexplainable—*not the result*. In other words, we can observe that the cancer is no longer present—an example of spontaneous remission. Once you make this observation you cannot just throw this information away because it cannot be measured using a quantitative or an objective material measurement system. In these cases, it is obvious the material research model does not adequately account for **all** the data being presented.

Systems of Interference is defined as *preconceived ideas which mitigate/manipulate information in a manner so that it super-imposes un-related data for inclusion or exclusion in an equation, experiment or reasoning process. This includes economic bias, pre-determined outcome of an experiment, anthropomorphic bias, racial prejudice, religious prejudice, social mores, political bias, group/mob mentality, gender bias, diploma mill indoctrination, or any other blind inclusion or exclusion of un-related data.*

Being aware of and understanding SI teaches you to be cognizant of how *you* filter information for recordation in your brain. *Please remember,* ***your information filter does not always allow*** *all the observed and available data to be utilized by you!* This happens to everyone who is not aware of their ego-based interpretation of reality. To make it easier to understand and remember, I call this a Reality Replication Template or (RRT) for short.

Any type of objective measuring methodology (quantitative methodology) is the scientific research community's preferred method for gathering data required to prove a hypothesis (I like it too!). However, as observed above, it only works with objective material forms of data. It stands to reason, once you begin observing data which cannot be accounted for using this type of "measuring stick approach", so to speak, other methods, including integrative methods, must be employed—like qualitative methodology—a way to collect and utilize invisible non-material information.

Qualitative Methodology

According to USC Library [4], "The word qualitative implies an emphasis on the qualities of entities and on processes and meanings that are not experimentally examined or measured [if measured at all] in terms of quantity, amount, intensity, or frequency. Qualitative researchers stress the socially constructed nature of reality, the intimate relationship between the researcher and what is studied, and the situational constraints that shape inquiry. Such researchers emphasize the value-laden nature of inquiry. They seek answers to questions that stress how social experience is created and given meaning. In contrast, quantitative studies emphasize the measurement and analysis of causal relationships between variables, not processes. Qualitative forms of inquiry are considered by many social and behavioral scientists to be as much a perspective on how to approach investigating a research problem as it is a method."

We need a way to account for the invisible and non-material observations. Qualitative methodology can be used to logically dissect data contained in a non-material observation, used in conjunction with material data, or as a separate stand-alone analogy. In other words, we will use at least two ways of collecting and measuring information in this book to insure all the information is accounted for.

I believe the best way to research any subject is to combine *all* the available data. (Note: If the definitions I am using seem unclear to you, please feel free to use any logical definition of qualitative methodology from any reasonable source you choose. It is always a good idea to examine and compare definitions since they employ linguistic trickery, manipulate your interpretation of knowledge, and your perceptions—academic indoctrination). To make this easier to understand, we can generally say that some observations can be measured, and some observations need to be extrapolated or reasoned. However, information that cannot be measured can be utilized if you apply logic to what you are looking at. This is especially true if there is a *material result* being presented during research. In your analysis of yourself, combining these two approaches will make complete sense and provide a more comprehensive way for you to understand how *you* become you.

A Systems Integration Approach

According to Techopedia [5], "System Integration is an IT or engineering process, or phase concerned with joining different subsystems or components as one large system. It ensures that each integrated subsystem functions as required. System Integration is also used to add value to a system through new functionalities provided by connecting functions of different systems."

As you have already seen, I adopted and adapted this same approach. It is utilized in our examination of self-healing and the different aspects of awareness. This system integration approach gives us a way to better understand examples of the material and non-material data we encounter in our everyday life and creates a more comprehensive and expanded analysis of *all* the available data.

Scientific evidence of any kind should never be omitted. Systems of interference of any kind should never be included. These observations are part of and support the overarching function of our entire quantum bio-system—not just its material expression. I believe humans exhibit an "awareness aspect" of themselves; they live in a world of images, feelings, and thought expressions that present themselves as photonic expressions in their minds and are experienced as an aspect of themselves in relation to their physical bodies. We will need to comprehend a basic understanding of the sciences involved in the building of the person we call *you*. Let us start with the following:

This is just background information using a few short definitions; we are *not* going to be teaching physics.

First, what is the difference between Newtonian physics and Quantum physics? Second, what is your individual specific reality with respect to the enigma that is you? Third, how do we incorporate this data to support "your interpretation" of the world around you--data which in turn supports your self-healing awareness and your RRT

According to Nikolas Scholz, M.S. Physics & Computational Science and Scientific Computing, Goethe University Frankfurt (2017) [6], "Newtonian physics assumes that everything in the universe has a specific and theoretically exactly specifiable position and momentum (and all the other crazier properties). In quantum physics this is dropped and found as relying on the action of specifying this property (called observation or measurement). Without measurement, anything we can say about something we don't know is statistical, and this truth (which is non-deniable for Newtonian physics too!) has interesting effects on the behavior of the object being measured, which is the craziness of quantum physics."

Doctor Amit Goswami states that a quantum understanding of *you* requires investigating the concept that "quantum waves of possibility can be collapsed into particles of reality through a process of evoking observation, with intention or measurement, by the observer." [7] This understanding, coupled with Reality Replication Templates, the Lock-on-Lock out principle and Systems of Interference allows us to create a useable template for self-healing and self-awareness.

Ok, we are done with this part of building your background information (If this is your first go around with quantum theory, relax and embrace the concept—this is an amazing perception of quantum reality). Niels Bohr said, "Those who are not shocked when they first come across quantum theory cannot possibly have understood it." Nevertheless, it is like moving to a new town and having everyone there give you directions that are meaningless unless you *already know some of what they are talking about*. For instance, you ask directions to the nearest grocery store. The person you ask tells you, "It is right next to where the old movie theatre used to be." You laugh because you have no idea where the old movie theatre used to be. So, you ask, "If you would be so kind, would you please give me an address and I will Google it on my phone." However, once you become acclimated to your new town and know some of the landmarks and history, *the directions you were given by that person make complete sense*. This is also true when investigating that quantum aspect of yourself called *you*. You will not only get a better understanding of yourself, but you will learn how to manipulate this aspect of yourself. This power allows you to control how you change your own awareness. Please remember, you already have this power. It is the *awareness of this power,* and your choice to use it, that provides an option for change.

Senses

All plants and animals have senses. (See partial list below). You and I use sensory information every day. Experiencing our senses gives us a subjective understanding of our environment. A subjective understanding means your *ego specific understanding*. This is observed for both plants and animals. Experiencing of our senses and the related analysis creates one's ego specific awareness which is combined with an individual ability to collect sensory data (it is important to remember that you are the ***only one*** who experiences sensory data in your environment in this manner). All sensory data is obtained through a process of utilizing your individual physical sensory mechanisms—sight, hearing, touch, taste, smell…19+ for humans and 22 + for plants (and the list is growing; see below). Also, note how many sensory mechanisms are the same for both plants and humans in this list. Please remember, your experience and understanding of this sensory data is not an all or nothing understanding. It is based on the "varying degrees" of your perception of the available knowledge gleaned from your environment and on the "varying degrees" of your individual specific sensory recordation capabilities; or how well your physical sensory receptors work during the process of collecting this data. Physical impairment or disease of sensory organs can affect how your data is received, perceived, and recorded in your brain. In addition to this, all these understandings are predicated on your Reality Replication Template. *Reality Replication Templates (RRT), coined by me, can be defined as the observed way humans develop their own individual specific versions of their self-awareness utilizing a subjective interpretation of their environment. These variables are different for everyone and mitigated by you.*

All humans hear sound differently, see their environment differently, experience taste differently, their sense of smell is different, their sense of time is different, their sense of proprioception is different, etc. You utilize and record data from the environment around you. You also interpret information from your non-material environment as "thought expressions" which can be used in conjunction with other material data (like smelling a rose or hearing a sound in your material environment and experiencing "thought expressions" in your non-material environment). You have probably noticed that I am using the word "your" a lot. This is done purposely to ingrain the concept that all this data is **yours and only yours**. This data is collected and perceived by your individual specific perception and recordation abilities. Sensory data exhibits both material and non-material properties; usually in combination. For instance, utilizing the sense of sight, you experience seeing a red rose. In a material observation of this rose you might notice it is red, has thorns, leaves, petals, roots, etc. However, a rose can also elicit an emotional response, like love, which is not a material construct or a visual observation; it is a feeling, an emotion or thought expression. A rose can also emit a scent (olfactory/smell) which elicits other physical and emotional responses, not to mention more thought expressions.

Sensory data is observed to continually combine to create quantum light expressions (pictures) or thought image expressions in your mind for recordation in your brain. All animals and plants use sensory data to define and analyze their environments. This creates a sense of themselves in relation to their environment and is observed to be part of a survival expression (yep, you do this too). This sense or awareness of yourself is an exciting part of investigating your own sensory awareness. Through this process you observe your ability to interpret sensory data and the way *you* filter it. This observation will also present an opportunity for you to use this data in a more effective and aware manner. *Once you become aware of anything, it creates options.* These options provide multiple choices (with awareness, you can interact, not just blindly react). In other words, more awareness creates more options to choose from. In this analysis, more options are better than fewer. This augmented awareness directly affects your self-healing awareness. Healing awareness is accomplished using intention to do so. Once you *intend* to augment your sense of awareness, it grows rapidly. This will create a new change—a quantum leap of your knowledge and of your perception of that knowledge.

LIST OF HUMAN AND PLANT SENSES

Humans

1. SIGHT
2. SMELL
3. TASTE
4. TOUCH
5. HEARING
6. PROPRIOCEPTION sense of relative position
7. EQUILIBRIOCEPTION sense of balance
8. NOCICEPTION' sense of nausea
9. THERMOCEPTION ability to sense heat
10. THIRST
11. HUNGER
12. EMPATHY
13. PAIN
14. TIME
15. AGENCY
16. FAMILIARITY
17. SELF AWARENESS
18. GRAVITY
19. MOTION

Plants

1. SIGHT
2. SMELL
3. TASTE
4. TOUCH
5. HEARING
6. PROPRIOCEPTION sense of relative position
7. EQUILIBRIOCEPTION sense of balance
8. THERMOCEPTION ability to sense heat
9. THIRST
10. PAIN
11. SELF AWARENESS
12. GRAVITY
13. MOTION
14. HUMIDITY
15. CHEMICAL SUBSTANCES
16. CHEMICAL GRADIENTS
17. REORIENTATION
18. MAGNETIC FIELDS
19. INFECTIONS
20. TISSUE DAMAGE
21. MECHANICAL PRESSURE
22. TIME

The environmental sensory data (19+) we collect are stand-alone information sources. However, they are often combined with other sensory information which allows the individual specific *you* to create and better support your interpretation of reality (your observations). This provides multiple perception interpretations (like the above stated example of seeing a red rose and smelling that rose; by combining sensory experiences of sight and smell, it creates an augmented understanding). After collecting this sensory data, you act upon this data in a manner consistent with what *you believe* to be real—your filtering mechanism. What you create is a Reality Replication Template (RRT). This is a subjective evaluation of the here and now created by you. All human life forms utilize RRTs. I will present evidence throughout this book which supports the logical conclusion that your reality is a collapse of quantum waves of possibility filtered by Systems of Interference related to what you intend to create—ultimately resulting in what I refer to as a (RRT) or your awareness of yourself-repeated over and over. This is explained below.

For instance, let us say you read a poem and you understood it to mean eternal love. The reading of the poem creates knowledge which can be stored in the brain and utilized later. The understanding of the poem is your perception. The "eternal love" conclusion is your individual specific awareness of the meaning of the poem. This can be simplified to mean Knowledge + Perception = Awareness or (K + P = A). However, the observation is humans *repeat* learning experiences over and over (humans are observed to be creatures of habit) and these learning experiences are inter-connected with all the other knowledge they have recorded in their brain. For instance, let us say after reading this poem you decide to read 100 more poems relating to love. Once completed, your knowledge of love poems has been augmented; you have read 101 poems. Your perception of love poems has been expanded; you now have more examples to choose from. Together, both the knowledge and perception interact and provide an integrated awareness of love poems. This in turn modifies your awareness of love poems. This observation is important to understand because all humans collect and interpret data in this manner.

We can use the following equation to make this easier to understand:

Knowledge = K

Knowledge repeated = K^r

Perception = P

Perception repeated = P^r

Awareness =A

Modified awareness =MA

Modified awareness repeated = MA^r

Reality Replication Template = RRT

Simplified equations can be helpful! I have listed and described what each abbreviation means with its verbal equivalent. However, if you do not want or like to utilize this type of brevity, I have described this information as follows: Knowledge + Perception = Awareness *ergo* **(K + P = A)** ***(Note, this is only theoretical).*** Knowledge affects perception and perception affects knowledge *ergo* **K - > P and P -> K** creating a feedback loop or circular concept. This can logically be interpreted to equate **(K <-> P** ∞) knowledge and perception affect each other endlessly. We can further observe that Knowledge (repeated) + Perception (repeated) will further modify one's awareness *ergo* if **(K <-> P)** then**, (**K^r **+** P^r **= MA)** and finally this modified awareness, if repeated, results in your reality replication template or **(**MA^r **= RRT)**. This means if you keep doing the same thing over and over you will create a subjective reality experience, an RRT, which is your preferred egoic experience of *you*—this is observed in *all* humans. (Yep, we all do it!) The main thing to remember is you are a creature that prefers repetitive experiences. Careful, it is a trap! Without awareness of this process you will do the same thing over and over without knowing why. This inhibits self-awareness.

Chapter 2

"The day science begins to study non-physical phenomena it will make more progress in one decade than in all the previous centuries of its existence."
—Nikola Tesla

"The man of science, who is not seeking for expression but for a fact to be expressed, merely studies nature as a dead language."—Henry D. Thoreau

Self-Healing

What is "healing"? Merriam Webster states [1], "to make free from injury or disease: to make sound or whole. B: to make well again: to restore to health. 2a: to cause (an undesirable condition) to be overcome. C: to patch up or correct (a breach or division) *heal* a breach between friends. Restore to original purity or integrity. To become free from injury or disease: to return to a sound state." All these definitions allude to a fragmented whole (the disease or breach) being normalized to its original complete state.

Before we continue with our study of self-healing and self-awareness, we should address a couple of misunderstood definitions confusing the word healing with the word curing. What is the definition of curing? Merriam Webster [2] states: "to restore to health, soundness, or normality, cured him of a rare blood disease. B: brings about recovery from a disease." This illustrates a similar but *notably different definition* from the word healing. **Healing alludes to a fragmented whole being normalized to its original complete state.** Whereas "curing" alludes to addressing a **specific ailment only**; it does not return the body and mind to its original healthy state or homeostasis. You can cure a patient of a specific ailment and they can still have one or more ailments that have not been addressed. I believe healing addresses the state of health and balance which exists in an entire live material and non-material human expression. Nevertheless, humans use the terms "healing" and "curing" interchangeably—and incorrectly. This affects your RRT.

How is healing accomplished? I believe healing is accomplished by an innate self-awareness response predicated on intelligent Photon Information Expressions which radiate from a live information field carrying information that appears to create, implement and direct a restorative bio-chemical, photonic and bio-electric response in living material or a mental body. Your self-awareness response detects imbalance (damage, disease, cognitive malfunction, bacterium intrusion, virus intrusion, etc.) in the physical and/or non-physical aspects associated with your material body or your mind. These "self-awareness responses" are thought expressions experienced in your mind that are collected and transmitted back and forth with this LIFE. To accomplish this, these thought expressions and awareness experiences use Photon Information Expressions (PIEs) which transport information embedded or encoded onto pictures or photonic images. In response, LIFE radiates back "healing directions" or maintenance instructions to the body, via the mind, which can create a state of balance and homeostasis. This "self-awareness response" coordinates a healing response that operates continuously in a waking or non-waking state. Self-healing is an intelligent, organized and complex process that promotes homeostasis and the continuation of the LIFE equation in a material body. It is important to note, this process is not an all or nothing response. Like many other aspects of the life experience, it exhibits varying degrees of a healing response that is predicated on one's physical and mental health. In other words, healing is dependent on how well your physical body can collect data from LIFE and how aware your mind is of this process—one must utilize a thought expression of "intent" to create change.

However, humans can support and augment this healing process by utilizing a self-generated thought expression—intent to do something. This is the first step. Intention originates from *you* and is an individual specific act of volition. What we can conclude from this is that **all healing and disease is affected by what you believe about yourself.** This creates a logical sequence of inter-connected healing responses in the physical and mental bodies. This self-healing response can be augmented or denigrated with self-direction through an intention to do so. This process of *intended self-healing* is an awareness belief or thought expression. The "thought expression" of "intention" is directed by you to interact with your physical body and your surrounding environment and logically interacts with other fields that flow into and out of your physical body (gravity, electricity, magnetism, etc.). The important thing to remember here **is a "thought expression" is an invisible, non-material observation which can create physical reality**.

I believe all healing is self-healing. Self-healing co-creates a healing collective experience—a projection of the individual specific interpretation of your healing experiences into a Total Information Continuum (TIC). This TIC is a database of information images and is part of the Live Intelligent Information Field Expression which directs the storing of thought image expressions (pictures).

As previously mentioned, it is my belief that this self-healing experience is directed by LIFE and utilizes Photon Information Expressions, extensions of LIFE, which radiate from and penetrate all live organisms. A live organism acts like an antenna or collector for this information field which radiates from this LIFE. In response, the live organism utilizes PIEs to upload information that is stored in a Total Information Continuum as data expressions (pictures of your collected data) and are analyzed by LIFE. In turn, LIFE radiates the proper healing responses back to the physical body using the same intelligent and organized PIEs. At this point *your* RRT or an environmental intrusion, or *both,* can augment or diminish this healing response. Another way of saying this is: pictures of information are uploaded to a database which is part of an intelligent, organized, living field expression that collects and analyzes information from all relative environments. The "field expression" then transmits healing information back to the material body (essentially an extension of itself) and directs the body to make the appropriate healing corrections if unimpeded. During this process, your RRT or your environment, or both, have a direct effect on how this data is used. Your beliefs and the experiencing of external data "trump" your existing DNA blueprint. This may help explain why there is no such thing as a set-in-stone interpretation of a genome. Your genome **can be, and is**, altered continuously by you or your environment(s) or a combination of these. I believe all life forms do this constantly and this can be likened to Herbert Froelich's model of a "coherent" organized field [3]. I also believe the awareness perception of the live field expression or database in turn *co-creates* what is required for all healing (maintaining the antenna or collector—you). This includes environmental healing, planetary healing, galaxy healing, and universe healing—a logical form of maintaining balance. In other words, when *your* physical and mental bodies become healthy and balanced, it affects all of existence (your gift to humanity and the universe; thanks!). Or the opposite effect can also become true! Human un-awareness and un-consciousness hinders the healing process and has the potential to destroy you, as well as the rest of life's expressions. Nevertheless, being unconscious of your innate quantum power facilitates change; and can cause problems. Unconsciousness can create deleterious effects on your RRT. Fortunately, once you become aware of yourself, you will discover warning signs or indicators that let you know when you are out of balance (you will *sense* insights of data). The observation that "something" is affecting your physical or mental body, whether it is disease or a psychological imbalance, will become apparent. This is not uncommon. However, the awareness of how this affects your ability to choose is uncommon and greatly impacts your awareness. This observation logically concludes that a conscious interconnection with all life is essential for our overall wellbeing.

As described here, all life is individual, interconnected and interdependent on this awareness. Everything we do affects everything else [4]. The individual specific *you* must intend to become aware to discover change. The blind alternative is manipulation or domination by Group Reality Replication Templates—you willingly or through manipulation go along with a group's interpretation of life's experiences rather than your own. You can choose to acquire a new perspective or new perception of self-awareness and self-healing which allows *you* to evolve in your material form, what I call psycho-biogenesis. This is easily accomplished (remember, you already do this) by using your abilities to collapse quantum waves of possibility into particles of reality by intending to create awareness. Intention to create this change is the first part of this process. If you want to know more about yourself or be more aware of your environment, ask this question of yourself: How do I become more aware of my ability to self-heal? Then just be quiet and the individual specific awareness will reveal itself! (Yep, it is that easy!) A common question I receive in response to this is, "What do you mean by 'it will reveal itself'?" In other words, the information field ***already exists.*** The observation is that you are immersed in this radiating field (like standing in sunshine). The field penetrates through you and radiates outward from within you. It affects a single live cell, 40 trillion live cells, or countless other expressions of our life experiences. You will discover this if you choose to. For example, discovering a field, like gravity, does not mean we invented it. It means our awareness perception finally noticed something that *already existed.* So, in using your "intent to discover" you will be able to access an already existing Live Intelligent Information Field Expression with your awareness. Once you experience this, you will understand what it means just like in the earlier example when you understand that "the grocery store is right next to where the old theatre used to be" only after you arrive at your destination. **Intend** to learn a new perspective, and the leap of awareness will occur. Your connection with your awareness of LIFE, which is manifested in, radiated to, and transmitted from your live material body, continues constantly until a death-transition occurs. Your mind is an invisible non-material quantum expression that communicates with your brain during the uploading and accessing of this stored information. As previously discussed, the mind instructs the brain to create new neurons to store data in the brain—a process known as neurogenesis. Although everyone does neurogenesis, few are aware of how to utilize this. Nor are they aware that the information transfer process is photonically encoded images. The *mind* can cause the brain to *create a material manifestation in the brain* (neurons) to store experiences observed within yourself and your environment(s). Think about this: You see it, you realized it as a "thought expression" in your mind and then this "thought image" is transformed into a *material reality.* From a non-material expression (invisible and not quantifiable), you can create a material expression that is quantifiable! Isn't this what the fifty or so Bibles said God did? Is God a quantum field expression which radiates through us? What else could God be? Nevertheless, it appears both LIFE and God are examples of quantum field expressions.

It is also my observation that this living innate healing awareness knows when and how to implement a change—which infers this healing awareness is alive and in constant contact with the body and mind. How else could this occur except through live interaction (See Chapter 7)? After a change is exhibited, you continue to modify and understand this awareness experience utilizing the previously mentioned processes: Knowledge repeated affects perception repeated which is stated as **(K^r <-> P^r).** Continuing forward, humans experience; Knowledge repeated + Perception repeated = Modified Awareness or **($K^r + P^r = MA$).**

Self-healing awareness can also address causes of medical conditions that have not been identified or been attributed an explanation of what is responsible (cause) for the malady. I believe successful healing responses from LIFE to a material body can be referred to as "quantum healing expressions" of data which can exhibit as a Miracle Cure, Spontaneous Remission, or a Placebo Effect.

Have you ever heard someone say, "We do not know what causes this disease"? This is a common and honest assertion given by medical professionals everywhere. However, the physical body, in conjunction with other intelligent non-material aspects of the human species, can access information from existing data fields and are constantly aware of these imbalances and disease. Your awareness or un-awareness affects your physical body's ability to receive information from this data field, a field I believe is constantly directing a healing response. Varying degrees of awareness mitigate the healing response and are directly affected by you and environmental intrusion.

Have you ever gone to your doctor and said, "There is something wrong with me"? This means *you* are aware of an imbalance; "something" is out of the norm. This "something" is a thought expression of awareness. How can you know "something" if it does not exist? You cannot. Trust the process of self-healing via awareness. I believe you should ALWAYS endeavor to augment this awareness. Learn what your physical and mental body's normal presentations are. Your body's immune system is continually eliminating pathogens and other intrusions experienced by your physical body and mind. The awareness of how this happens originates from your environment and/or yourself. Your ability to utilize self-healing constantly addresses imbalances (maintenance and balance of your physical and mental body expressions) of your health unless interrupted or diminished by conscious or unconscious choices made by you or an external intrusion from your environment—like toxins, bacterium, viruses, etc.

Most manifestations of disease are observed to be directly related to non-support of the immune system, which means it is not only poor diet and sleep, lack of exercise, intrusions of toxins, cognitive imbalances, etc. that inhibit (physical and mental) health. It is your invisible and non-material belief system of yourself or your RRT that supports or impedes the process of self-healing. The mind affects the body and the body affects the mind. The mind and body can *only* be separated by a death-transition.

I believe if you think you are sickly, you create a corresponding thought expression of yourself. You collapse the possibility of being "sickly" into reality! This "thought expression" is physically recorded in your brain (neurogenesis) per your mind's instructions. You literally create this state of mind! It is your self-identification (ego interpretation) or RRT which continues to support this belief. **This "thought expression" cannot exist if you do not create it.** If you think you catch the flu every year, it is you who is *trying* to achieve this goal. Many people I share this with say, "Well, it's the truth. Look at my medical records for the last seven years!" They forgot they did not *always* have the flu. It is you who collapsed these quantum waves of possibilities into particles of reality, and filtered the information from your environment which supported this conclusion (be careful of what you wish for; quantum possibilities allow *anything* to be collapsed into reality). However, I am happy to say, by choosing to be aware of this process you now have the "choice" to change. Why would you choose to be ill? In general, this would not make any logical sense. However, only you can answer this (maybe it is your mechanism for interfacing with society)? Nevertheless, this is a reality created by you. I have met hundreds of "professional patients" blind to who they are. However, some of us can see them. Ralph Waldo Emmerson is attributed with saying something like, "Who you are speaks so loudly I can't hear what you are saying." Why would someone choose to be ill or want to experience a death-transition? Self-awareness gives you the ability to support and heal your entire existence. You no longer need to be trapped in an unconscious RRT cycle. Your goal, if you choose to experience it, is to achieve and augment your ability for self-healing and self-awareness. You can achieve a balanced state of health for every aspect of your awareness—an awareness which affects *everything else*. It is important to remember you can choose to change, or you can choose to do the same thing. It is *you* who chooses! **There is no right or wrong, only levels of awareness.**

Chapter 3

"Man knows that he springs from nature and not nature from him. This is an old and very primitive knowledge."—Loren Eiseley

"...Awareness of "how" you obtain and process information, is just as important as the information you are collecting." —Dr. G. Munger

How YOU Affect Everything

Now that we have a better understanding of ourselves and how we got this way, we can address how your everyday life experiences become part of a "human species collective" of information. The human species continually radiates and shares their individual specific life experiences with all fields identified in the universe and each other. This is a collective of all the information the human species experiences as a field of photonic data" (images with information attached) located in what I call the Total Information Continuum. The TIC is the data collection and transmission aspect of the original and eternal intelligent Live Information Field Expression (LIFE) we spoke of earlier.

It is a common observation that humans share their perspective about life with other humans. This can only be done using their Reality Replication Templates (RRTs). We are constantly accessing various information that we collect from our environments (local and non-local). The information we collect is attached to Photon Information Expressions which radiate to and from you constantly. This is experienced as a "field" emanating to and from our physical bodies and is directly connected to the universal Live Intelligent Information Field Expression. I believe your data stream is stored in this field expression's database. A brain-like data repository—a crude comparison.

It appears all live data is collected, positive or negative, and is constantly being uploaded to this TIC or the brain-like repository of LIFE (Yep! You are already doing this). It is important to remember your PIEs are an integral part of the circular concept of LIFE. Through this process, data is transmitted from every living organism to this infinite universal field which I nicknamed "LIFE" to make it easier to remember. Due to the ambiguity associated with our individual specific abilities to gather and interpret information in our environment, we should always remember: **Awareness of "how" you obtain and process information is just as important as the information you are collecting**.

Humans and other life forms constantly create who they are with the help of LIFE, PIEs, LoLo effect (lock-on and lock-out) and RRTs—the expressions of your subjective reality experience.

The current assertion made by the scientific community states humans update the data in their genes until the moment their body recycles (death-transition). I believe part of this death-transition is the final emission our individual specific sensory data back into the Total Information Continuum, a database of holographic images of your life experience. I believe this is a continuous flow of living photonic data. The "Live Intelligent Information Field Expression" is present in all living species and is experienced using its extension, or their Photon Information Expressions. This LIFE can also be referred to as the original consciousness, or God field, if you will. It is invisible, and only detectable using logical extrapolation from our subjective observations. Nevertheless, the observation of a PIE manifested in a physical body is easily and logically concluded by observing a death-transition occurrence (a live field of PIEs leaving a physical body).

The degree of access one has to this database of information in the LIFE field is contingent on your awareness and desire to use intention to access it. (Note: If you do not know it exists, how can you access it?). Sometimes, as Madeleine L'Engle is quoted as saying, "Some things have to be believed to be seen." We constantly add our individual specific self to this existing database, consciously or un-consciously until a death-transition occurs.

Quantum awareness is not exclusively a human awareness It belongs to all life. It appears all life forms can receive or transmit information to this field. Species that access this data do so utilizing their individual specific awareness and data filtering capabilities. For instance, a common garden spider knows how to weave a web in a geometric pattern. Where did the spider acquire this information, and how? Many humans exalt themselves and believe they are the superior intelligence on earth and are not affected or subject to a superior intelligence or. A general observation of humans reveals they appear to believe and exhibit an ego centric interpretation which elevates them to the highest example of a life form. If a God or a Quantum Continuum were logically included in this ego centric analysis, then this assumption would be flawed. Remember, only your interpretation or perception of data is considered or analyzed by you (it is important to remember this). This is a classic example of a Reality Replication Template, Systems of Interference and LOLO effect. Humans create not only their own Reality Replication Template, but they also create a Reality Replication Template that others of the same species can align with as a ***group***. These examples of Group Reality Replication Templates (religions, politics, diploma mill indoctrination, gender bias, and unfortunately many more) promote a herd mentality or agreed upon awareness. This can be problematic when new information is presented to these GRRTs because all the data being presented is filtered and interpreted to support the GRRT observation *agreement*. Consequently, some information is not processed nor considered! Nevertheless, the sound waves or vibrations carrying this information are observed to strike the tympanic membrane in your ear (What!). It is you who chooses to *hear* it or not. As discussed earlier, these groups listen, evaluate, and accept or reject any new data. If the data is accepted, it resonates with the agreed upon reality of the group—literally. If this data is not selected to be included in this group, it is rejected. The important thing to remember here is your data filtering prohibits you from including this data; it is *not even experienced.* However, this acceptance or rejection is not observed to be predicated on the data being factual or un-supported. The observation is the collective awareness of this Group Reality Replication Template is a generally accepted awareness, an agreed upon mind awareness definition and it *resists* being altered. This can be an awareness that is considered positive or negative (it can be a group that helps their community, or it can be a group with mob mentality). This type of awareness is enormously powerful and persuasive. Please remember, this type of group awareness is not necessarily a factual awareness. **Historically, it has taken people who do not agree with a species collective interpretation to create change**. Our past experiences show that change is exceedingly difficult to implement when this equation exists. The old saying, "Everybody knows" or "Most of the universities say…" usually "trumps" new awareness and new knowledge regardless of the proof presented. This state of invincible ignorance incorporates Systems of Interference—creating an almost impenetrable Reality Replication Template shield.

However, aware and conscious forms of a Group Reality Replication Templates are considered beneficial to all life forms—like groups forming to clean the earth's air, water, soil, regulate social interactions, etc. These GRRTs can create global cooperation and understanding.

All GRRTs are a choice predicated on filtered data and awareness.

It is interesting to note some examples of Reality Replication Templates are also Systems of Interference. Group Reality Replication Templates are evidence of an incomplete and ignorant interpretation of information which are exhibited within these Group Reality Replication Template experiences. These examples do not have to make any logical sense (and seldom do). They require a great deal of analyzing to discover how they are formed in the first place. They are perplexing, at best.

Self-awareness and self-healing can offer a template for healthy change. However, it is wise to be aware of the many examples of "templates" that promote a different agenda and are contrary to creating a balanced self and life. Some examples include economic bias, pre-determined outcome of an experiment, anthropomorphic bias, racial prejudice, religious prejudice, social mores, political bias, group/mob mentality, gender bias, diploma mill indoctrination, etc. You will undoubtedly benefit from an awareness of Systems of Interference (SI) while creating your existence. You are the chief architect of *you*; leave SI out of your creation.

In general, the human species wants to be "like" all the other humans—even if being like all the rest is illogical or exhibits an insane herd or mob mentality. This observation is even more reason to self-heal and acquire the awareness of the all-important, one in 7.7

billion; you. Please remember, support your self-awareness. It is the key to universal awareness. Our interconnectedness ***is accomplished one person at a time***.

This information is included to illustrate how known factors which mitigate your existence are unknown to most people. These factors affect your self-healing awareness and your very existence. All that is required to change these factors is a quantum leap of your perception of *self*. Remember, this is a process you already do. Choose to be the person you always knew you were—you will never be dissatisfied. When you become aware of your ability to create quantum leaps into new realities, you will experience continued opportunity for growth.

Chapter 4

"...Self-awareness is a choice."—Dr. G. Munger

"The search for truth is more precious than its possession" —Gotthod Lessings dictum

A New Perspective

It was another hot summer night and time for my younger brother, Tommy, and I to go to bed. I was eight years old and living in a ranch style house with creaking wooden floors in a farming community in California. In those days we did not have air conditioning. We made do with a swamp cooler. However, the "swamp cooler" was in our living room. This left us with the only other available option—ventilation. We took advantage of the cross-breezes created by opening windows.

After baths, pajamas, and "stalling" (I did not like having to go to bed when I was younger) I could see the expression on my Mother's face was changing. The usual threats of "go to sleep or else" were getting very close to "or else". So, my brother and I took the "hint" and begrudgingly went to bed.

This night my Mother was ironing clothes in our bedroom with the windows open. My brother and I liked this because it gave us more time to be awake due to the bedroom light being on, while we pretended to be asleep. Nevertheless, we both eventually fell asleep.

Hours later, I awoke to the sound of a creaking floorboard near the door to my bedroom. As I looked in the direction of the door, I realized what was making this creaking sound—it was a burglar, and he was in my room! Even with the lights off, I could see the outline of the burglar due to the ambient light creeping in around and under my bedroom door from the light left on in the hallway. I felt my heart speed up and thump against my chest. I was terrified, and I did not know what to do. I could see the burglar's head, arms, and legs. He was just standing there waiting. But, waiting for what? I quietly woke my brother; whose bed was next to mine. In a whispering voice, I said, "Tommy wake-up". Sluggishly, my brother woke up. Trembling, I pointed to the burglar. Tommy also became scared and whimpered a little very quietly. I used a yelling whisper and said, "Shut up he is going to hear us." Still whispering, I told my brother, "Do not worry, I have plan. We will both jump on the burglar. We will scream and yell for Dad, and Pop will finish him off."

Tommy said, "No, I can't!"

I said, "I can't do this without you! Look, he is going to hurt us. We need to do something. I will hit him high and you kick him in the balls. Dad will do the rest."

Reluctantly, Tommy agreed. One, two, three we attacked the burglar! Within seconds our bedroom light went on (parents know the sound of *real* emergency screams and crashing sounds—they reacted quickly) and my *entire family* was standing there in their underwear. I was astonished as I looked around the bedroom and saw there was no burglar—only the ironing board which my brother and I had just destroyed.

My Mother had folded the ironing board to stand upright and hung the ironed clothes on it. The long sleeve shirts were on hangers near the top and under these were pants which hung down lower towards the bottom of the ironing board near the floor—my burglar. To my embarrassment and relief, I realized I was wrong and there was no burglar. A new reality replaced my old awareness—a quantum leap.

What transpired in the above *true* story is known as a quantum leap of awareness. Originally, a quantum leap referred to when electrons orbiting around an atom jumped, leapt, or teleported to another orbit.[1] However, all things change. A definition of a quantum leap has been linguistically augmented to also include: "Any sudden or discontinuous change."[1] This definition of a quantum leap refers to a greater understanding, a better understanding of information in a manner which *prohibits* utilizing the old data.

This new reality displaced my old reality and I would never be able to believe the old burglar reality again. My new awareness was irrevocable! However, before I experienced this new awareness, I believed whole heartedly that the "burglar" version of my awareness was real. Real enough to convince my brother of this "truth". The terror was real. My reaction was real. I did not think for a second that I was wrong.

Achieving a quantum leap is something *all of us already do.* However, most people are not aware of this ability. To illustrate this further, I will provide another example of an everyday irreversible quantum leap which prohibits you from using the previous information once the quantum leap has been experienced. You have probably already experienced this.

For instance, have you ever heard the lyrics to a song and thought the words being sung were something other than what they really were? Later, sometimes years later, you run across the original sheet music/lyrics or other reliable source and exclaim, "Wow, I always thought what was being sung was, (insert your misinformation here)". Once you know the actual lyrics you *cannot* go back to your original perception. To do so would be illogical, even insane. This is a quantum leap of awareness. The pertinent point to remember here is you continued to use faulty information until the quantum leap of understanding was experienced. This is an example of a Reality Replication Template, the Lock-on Lock-out principle and Systems of Interference which we discussed earlier. How many other concepts, lyrics, understandings, including your health awareness definitions, do you believe that could benefit from a quantum leap?

People use faulty information a lot when evaluating their state of health. They make unfounded realizations or, even worse, they let others do it for them. They just "rubber stamp" the conclusion, like my brother did in the above-mentioned story. This is especially powerful when someone you *trust* tells you about a pending health danger or possibly a disease that could cause a death-transition experience.

Now, apply the new quantum self-healing awareness illustrated above to one of your memories or medical conditions. Is your memory or medical condition a "burglar" or an "ironing board"? What is needed to turn on your light? Think back on any perceptions of knowledge you experienced in the past. While you were reading the above examples, were you *aware* they were definitions of a quantum leap? My examples, and more to the point your examples, indicate the importance of further investigation into how quantum leaps affect your self-awareness and self-healing. Please take a few minutes to remember other examples, as this will be instructive to your understanding of a quantum leap. Also, remember that self-reflection is important, as it will provide examples which illustrate all this quantum theory mumbo jumbo is *real* and is constantly being programmed by *you*. Remember, self-awareness is a choice.

The above examples are already creating "new awareness" constructs in your mind for you to consider. These are insights into your individual specific awareness and how to modify your state of perception and knowledge. Additionally, these awareness perceptions are beginning to augment *your* understanding of self-healing.

There are thousands and thousands of examples of quantum leaps of perception evident in medicine. They can be observed as a miracle cure, spontaneous remission, placebo effect or heightened health awareness. These are examples of a healing awareness perception. The important point to remember here is, as previously mentioned, it does not mean you do not remember the previous medically (or other) inhibited awareness, but that you can no longer logically or sanely base decisions on this old information. This awareness, or lack thereof, determines the effectiveness of your ability to self-heal. To paraphrase Henry Ford, "If you think you *can*, you're right. If you think you *can't* you're right.".

Remember, self-healing is not an all or nothing awareness. It is a self-healing awareness consisting of varying degrees of knowledge and perception. The more aware you become, the more options you will have at your disposal to facilitate, support and augment self-healing—a significant advantage. Awareness is different for everyone, and is predicated on our previously discussed Reality Replication Template, the Lock-on Lock-out principle and your individual specific examples of Systems of Interference.

Awareness is further augmented by learning how the mind and brain interact to combine and record your interpretation of information (Photonic Encoding). This will be elaborated on in our next chapter, "…and the truth shall set you free." [2]

Chapter 5

"All physical phenomena, from the largest to the smallest, are described as frequencies of discrete angular occurrence of intimately contiguous but physically discontiguous events." Buckminster Fuller

"...A non-audible sound experienced in your mind does not vibrate, nor is it quantifiable as a material observation as stated in science's standard definition."— Dr. G. Munger

Photonic Encoding:

(New Revelations on How the Mind and Brain Work)

As I emerge from a restful slumber, my day starts out with immersion into my local sensory environment. I absolutely love the quiet of early morning. It is the perfect time to meditate and be grateful. I get to experience the sun rise; it never grows old. I hear birds singing and all life is waking up. I feel the floor under my feet and the temperature of the air against my skin. I stumble into the kitchen to prepare a cup of Chai tea and breathe in the wonderful aroma it emits. I sip my tea while planning out my day (I am happier than thirteen hippies and a big dog). Seamlessly, I combine and experience up to 19 known types of sensory data, both consciously and unconsciously—this my reality.

I was taught that the sensory data you experience in your environment is recorded directly into your brain via your senses. For instance, once you hear a sound or experience the vibrations striking the tympanic membrane in your ear, this "sound" is interpreted and directed to your brain for recordation. However, this is not the observation. Sensory information is utilized by your mind and recorded in your brain in a different manner. It is not what you have learned in school. What happens is a process I coined called: Photonic Encoding. As I previously mentioned, new information is difficult to impart to Reality Replication Templates. We are all subject to our own interpretation of our knowledge—you and I are no exception. The important difference is being aware that you do this.

Photonic Encoding (PE) can be described as a process in which the mind and physical brain of humans, or a neural-like-network (NLN) in other organisms, coordinate the retrieval and recording of sensory data to and from the brain or NLN, as photonic images (holograms) and not the actual sensory data input experienced (with the exception of the sense of sight). This is easily observed. This *variation* of sensory data is represented as a hologram or a series of pictures which are imprinted, superimposed, or encoded with information to create a memory for future retrieval from the brain. This is accomplished by utilizing an intent to do so—a "thought expression of intention". This intention expression is self-generated by you and is programmed as part of your Reality Replication Template.

Sensory Data Conversion Equation for Photonic Encoding (PE)

SD = Sensory Data

SD^r = Sensory Data Repeated

PE = Photonic Encoding

PED = Photonically Encoded Data

M = Memory

M^r = Second recordation sensory data Repeated

Photonic encoding of human memory consists of the everyday information you have collected and experienced. This is a material representation of sensory data perceived by the mind and recorded in the brain. I believe once the sensory data is collected, it is then superimposed or combined with light (photonic frequencies of 430 – 770 Hz of the electromagnetic spectrum of radiation—pictures). Information encoded photons are recorded in the physical brain as memory (sensory data plus photonic encoding equals memory **(SD + PE = M)**. This is a departure from the notion that sensory data is directly imputed into the brain [1] or a neural-like networking system in other organisms as the actual sensory data being experienced. Nevertheless, when the same sensory data, or similar sensory data, is experienced, or recorded again, it is combined and utilized with previously recorded sensory data (memory) which were recorded using photonic images. These images are variations and not the original sensory data. This data is combined with the retrieved data from the physical brain in a form that is recognizable as a holographic mental construct (an image). *However, the image perceived in the mind is not the original sensory data.* This event is experienced relative in the flow of time as the here and now. Ergo, utilizing previously encoded sensory data (memory) with the same type of new experienced sensory data results in real time recognition and recall after which the mind and brain instantaneously re-encodes the new sensory data into another memory. This is a Reality Replication Template of the same or similar sensory experience. Sensory data repeated + previously encoded data + memory = the memory repeated. The important thing to remember is: *None of the original sensory data is present during the recalling of a sensory memory.* What is observed is a photonic image, a variation (see examples below). This new assertion demands an expanded definition of various sensory data and an elaboration on the photonic encoding process.

Hold on to your hat, here we go!

A new function of photonic expressions is observed to exist. This new function exhibits environmental sensory data being experienced in the mind as being combined with photons (imprinted and encoded with data) for recordation and retrieval from the human brain. One of the obvious sensory exceptions to this is our sense of sight or “visible light” (390 to 700 nm, or frequencies of 430-770 Hz) in the electromagnetic spectrum of radiation, EMS.

According to Google and others, this is a relatively thin and narrow frequency band in the vicinity of 430-770 Hz of the entire electromagnetic spectrum of light.[3] It is important to note, visible light is not required to be encoded due to it already being comprised of photons. However, the image still presents itself for a "subjective interpretation" as part of your quantum modified awareness experience. It extrapolates the associated information which creates your Reality Replication Template. In other words, you still interpret images you see and make your own decision on how, or if, you want to record them in long or short-term memory.

For instance, if we use the sense of hearing in regard to sound waves, as an example of photonic encoding, we experience a phenomenon I coined as *non-audible audio* or sound that does not correspond to the scientific definition of sound.[4] Non-audible audio is experienced when intention is used to recall a memory of a sound wave sensory experience. **During this process, a photonic representation of the sound is retrieved instead of the actual sound wave vibration**. This can be evidenced by the reader of this chapter using their own intent to recall a particular sound (one can use any sound vibration, but recalling a high decibel (loud) sound will make quantifying much easier; your choice) and then place an electronic stethoscope or more sophisticated sound amplification device on the scalp to see if the recorded sound is present (NOTE: I have done this experiment multiple times and have **never** observed sound to be present). If sound were present, you would "experience a vibration or audible wave". [5] What is apparent is that the sound is not re-created using the currently accepted definition of sound. Instead a photonic image or holographic image(s) is recalled which directly corresponds to the recordation of this sound event—a variation. **A "non-audible" sound experienced in your mind does not vibrate, nor is it quantifiable as a material observation as stated above in science's standard definition**. This logically insists on an encoding or imprinting of sound data which is *superimposed* or combined with *something else* for recordation in the human brain. What we know is the recalled image is a photonic expression—a picture or image in your mind. This provides a logical connection to photons. Photonic encoding by the mind to the brain during the recording or recalling of a memory is a logical extrapolation. In this example, the process superimposes soundwave data upon a photonic image. This is a variant sound experience which cannot be heard by anyone except the individual experiencer. This variation or imprinted photonic version of the sound experience is different from the currently acceptable scientific definition of sound. It exhibits properties previously unknown and which have not been investigated qualitatively or quantitatively. Nor has this been acknowledge by scientific investigation until now.

If you are thinking and/or talking to yourself no one hears this conversation except you (You gotta be grateful for this!). This "thought experience" takes place in your mind, a non-material or non-local construct, and no one hears what you are thinking. This conversation or thought process of hearing your voice does not occur in the conventional sense, nor does it comply with the current definition of sound. However, it is perceived *exactly as your version* of the original sound experience (It should be noted that when most people hear a recording of their own voice for the first time, they do not recognize it—try this yourself). This observation is significant in that the data is perceived as accurate, but it does not actually utilize a specific sensory (hearing) perception nor comply with accepted scientific definitions of sound waves. We must conclude new aspects of sound waves and the EMS are present. I believe sensory data combined with photonic frequencies needs to be considered during this analysis.

Merriam-Webster's definition of sound [6] is too vague and does not include cognitive phenomena or the non-local data associated with the collection and storage of environmental data. Due to the exclusion of the above stated observations from science's current definition, I am required to augment the definition of "sound" to **include** the cognitive awareness and quantum experience of "non-audible audio" and its direct inter-connection and dependence upon photonic images to record and transmit sensory data associated with sound waves.

Photonic encoding of sensory data for retrieval from the human brain is a phenomenon which is very different from the material quantification experienced as the actual sensory input (vibration). Conscious intent, a thought expression concept, utilizes a "new variation" of the sensory data experience (encoded photons) to recall the sensory data. It decodes the existing data stored in the brain. Together, the mind and brain recognize this "vibration" as a memorized sound wave that has combined the sensory data of sound with photonic images and is experienced in a visual form (you see a picture associated with the sound experience, *rather than hear it*). This method of sensory recordation of data is experienced by all humans (unless impaired) and is pertinent to our discussion of collapsed quantum waves of possibility into particles of reality using intent, observation, or measurement. It is also observed to exhibit a non-material construct or awareness which facilitates this ability. The following is another example:

Please try this experiment too. It can be done with any sensory data, we just need to modify the testing equipment to test for the sensory data being selected (Non-odorous olfactory, non-tactile touch, non-present taste, etc.). For this example, think of an odor or scent. Let us say it is Thanksgiving and your mother is baking an apple pie. Let us assume you love apple pie and the scent it emits during the baking process. Now, remember this event. What comes to mind? Is there an actual odor present? No. What is present is an individual specific *holographic* representation of the sensory (olfactory) expression recorded in your brain. The actual sensory data of an aroma has been encoded into a photonic image which I coined as "non-odorous olfactory". Additionally, this non-odorous olfactory can only be experienced by you. Now, let us say later you go somewhere where there is an actual apple pie baking. Your sensing (olfactory) of the actual aroma in your material world triggers a memory of an individual specific *image* of an apple pie baking and you can identify this picture as associated with the aroma of a baking apple pie. Experiencing an actual sensing event decodes the holographic images to identify the aroma as that of a baking pie in your recorded memory. This variation is recalled as an image(s) of your experience. It is recognized and decoded. It provides a picture of the actual pie baking (your individual specific picture) as a holographic picture from your memory and then extrapolates the data experienced as recognition of the scent of an apple pie.

The process from encoding to decoding only happens in an actual or similar odor experience. Once again, the important point to remember is the memory never exhibits an odor/scent as being present (How could it?). Now, think of a scent, smell, or odor. While you are thinking about it, have someone assist you in this experiment that has heightened olfactory, or employ the scientific equipment of your choice to measure this. Ask them if they can smell the scent you are thinking (I would make it an easy one, like the time you were sprayed by a skunk; if that were present the whole room would be toxic. However, it is your choice). Decide for yourself and make your own observation experience of your own experiment. I have repeated this experiment numerous times with the result being no aroma being detected. Remember, you only experience the aroma/scent as a holographic image or photonically encoded data. **You do**

not actually have any of the actual scent physically present in your brain as a chemical. This same result can be experienced using any sensory data, except photonic images, as they are already photonic expressions. (NOTE: There is always an exception, I believe you can experience photonic sensory data (an insight or thought expression) due to it being a photonic expression experience, like the example of my "sudden knowing".

As previously discussed, the mental construct, or the mind, is a non-material expression which utilizes photonic images or holograms of stored sensory data. These are utilized alone or in conjunction with your knowledge and perception. This is experienced simultaneously when "intent" is initiated and mitigated by your own individual specific knowledge and perception. This sequence of cognitive experiences creates subjective awareness or individual specific awareness within the mind of the person. Photonic sensory data is observed to be recorded as a perception of a holographic image and is mitigated by Systems of Interference and the individual specific data filtering processes of the person observing the holographic experience (RRT). It is interesting to note that the recall of photonic images by humans are observed to be completely individual specific, yet identifiable as a "generalized experience" by any observer who has experienced the same sensory data. **This demonstrates the existence of new a system (or the re-discovering an**

old) of collecting information based on photonic encoding—photonic information expressions.

I have included the results of a supplemental experiment (See Chapter 15, Subjective Memory Experiment) which required a group of randomly selected people to respond to a request to draw a picture of a tree. This was the only information they received. The results of the drawings submitted were all different. I submit these images for your review. These images are examples of individual specific representations of their awareness of recalled information for the purpose of drawing a tree. The significance of this is that all the above-mentioned images of trees are different, but all are *recognized* by other humans as being acceptable images of trees. It does not matter whether it is a work of art or a lolly-pop tree. It does not matter that one is a pine tree and the next a palm tree, and the next an elm tree, and the next your own personal example of a tree. They represent individual specific subjective data evaluation of a recalled memory. This is a process which utilizes photonic images, or holograms, as a "generalized method" and understanding for retrieval of encoded photonic sensory data.

These data become even more individual specific when we add the participants' artistic ability to draw a tree into the experiment, or lack thereof, to replicate what *they remember* as a picture of a tree. The emphasis here is that all their answers to the instruction to "Draw a picture of a tree" are <u>different</u>, yet <u>all are considered correct!</u> As mentioned, this is supportive of the existence of another type of memory recordation and retrieval for data expressions utilizing an "information field" (Total Information Continuum) which collects data attached to photonic image expressions. I believe this "field" is accessed by all living organisms—we are immersed in it. Living organisms constantly augment and change this field. The Subjective Memory Experiment illustrates this phenomenon. The recordation and retrieval of data from this "Total Information Continuum" is observed to use photonic images (PIEs) to record and transmit data. I believe photons are a good choice to record data on as they do not appear affected by entropy, annihilation, or the flow of time. Additionally, this phenomenon appears to happen in either an "awakened state of awareness" or a "sleeping state of awareness". This observation may partially account for the dream state rapid eye movement (REM) that humans' experience while sleeping; the results of which commonly exhibit ambiguous, illogical and inane imagery (I believe this is due to receiving **snippets** of holographic images from various EMS frequencies not specifically generated by you, but received by you while sleeping (like turning the dial on a radio or TV quickly to scan the available stations that are broadcasting). This data field (TIC) is accessed utilizing an altered and relaxed state of consciousness (more on this later).

These observations propose a clearer understanding of human sensory data storage and retrieval from the brain. Photonic encoding of sensory data exhibits how photons or holographic images record sensory data for retrieval from the physical brain by the mind and are experienced using Photon Information Expressions which are extensions of LIFE.

This observation is evidence that the phenomenon of photonic encoding is a non-local intelligent Live Information Field Expression that instantaneously and intelligently encodes and de-codes sensory data in conjunction with the mind and human brain or NLN in other living organisms. This is an example of the sensory data processing present in sapient humans' and, logically, would also be present in sapient and sentient examples of other living organisms in the animal or plant kingdom that fit this same definition.

The above paragraph provides observations that act like a bridge between the Plant and Animal kingdoms and are pertinent to understanding plants and their role regarding humans. (See Chapters 9 & 10). Plants are supplements to the self-healing process (Humans have been using them for millennia). To illustrate this better, I have chosen an example of the bumble bee orchid to be examined from a human perspective (see Chapter 11, The Bumble Bee Orchid (Ophrys-Bombyliflora). The study of the memory aspect of the bumble bee orchid would include using photonic encoding as a possible way in which plants' record sensory data. I provided examples that exist in humans, but not in plants. However, it is important to note the scientific community is still unclear about where sensory information is stored in plants and, specifically, the bumble bee orchid. Additionally, I am unable to perform the same type of testing that I performed on humans for obvious reasons (I cannot orally communicate with plants). I hypothesize the bumble bee orchid also uses a similar neuro-like network process (probably located in their root system). It is my belief, with the evolution of technology, science will undoubtedly quantify this observation in plants soon.

Photonic encoding is pertinent to creating your Reality Replication Template and gives one insight into your ability to self-heal. This points us toward a quantum understanding of life itself. Part of this understanding is relating old data to new data and trying to understand how the old data was created. Auras and other light emanations can help us reflect on this (pun intended).

Chapter 6

"The wide dispersion of brain areas involved in imagery—especially visual imagery—indicate the importance of imagery to the survival of the species"— Joanne Actherberg

"...according to this study photons are emitted from all living things."—Dr. G. Munger

Auras and Emanations are Photonic Expressions

The following chapter is a fun and thought-provoking analysis. Review this data and start making your own interpretations—write them down for later use. Remember, we are locating and building *your* reality, not replicating mine.

Bioluminescence and other forms of light emissions from live organisms are evident throughout nature [1]. Most examples of bioluminescent emanations are easily seen by humans using their unaided eyes (Fireflies, jellyfish, algae, etc.). However, being able to see auras emanating from humans appears to be an uncommon ability.

An aura is a translucent subtle radiation that surrounds the human body or other objects. Auras have been attributed to everything from spiritual or religious emanations to hallucinations and psycho-visual impairment. Until recently, auras were thought to be scientifically explainable and attributable to physical and psychological disorders, and not a result of the body emitting light, or the electromagnetic emanations commonly depicted in early Christian era paintings and manuscripts.

As with most things, change is inevitable. In a joint research effort conducted at Tohoku Institute of Technology and Kyoto University in Japan, scientists have discovered that humans emit light. This light is very weak, a thousand times less than most humans can see. However, this experiment shows that light **is** emitted by humans with the strongest emissions observed to come from the head. According to "Science Blog", a United Kingdom based internet periodical, "Humans glow in the dark." [2] Nevertheless, it is pertinent to our understanding of photonic encoding to note "…early Christian era paintings depict auras" and or the emanations mentioned above. If the emanations are too weak to be seen by the human eye, why did ancient artists paint them? This alludes to an individual specific ability to perceive these emanations (frequencies) and possible physiological differences with respect to the structure of the eyes of people who can see auras. Additionally, the influence of their Reality Replication Templates could predispose them to this ability.

Two teams of Japanese scientists using ultra-sensitive cameras revealed that humans emit tiny amounts of light. As previously mentioned, these emissions are extremely weak. ***According to this study, photons are emitted from all living things.*** [3] Why? It is interesting to note that the photon emissions are significantly stronger around the face, forehead and neck, the part of the human body purported to emit auras. Why does the human body collect and store photons for emission (The body must use them, or why collect them)? What tissues store these photons? Are they used for cellular communication? Photonic encoding? **Why** are photons mainly concentrated in the face, forehead, and neck? How are photons emitted? If photons are emitted by *all* living organisms, doesn't this conclude photons are necessary elements of the life equation? This observation has been omitted in our definitions of auras and life? This means humans utilize photons as a necessary part of their life equation. These new data pose the question: Are photons a living organism's inter-connectedness, a commonality observed in *all* life forms that use Photonic Information Expressions to communicate with all available bio-organisms?

We know photons mainly enter through our eyes and skin—two extremely complex organs. Why? The images taken by these scientists are the first ever examples of human bioluminescence. Could photonic expressions be the *key* to developing a truly universal language; one that can communicate with all living organisms? Bridge all languages? I believe, yes. Remember, all languages use images.

I believe the universal Live Intelligent Information Field Expression, via its "extension" a Photon Information Expression, is already using photonic expressions (encoding) to superimpose and record sensory data (See Chapters 7) to the human brain. Is the answer to universal communication staring us in the face? This field of information expressions will have answers to questions that pre-date human existence.

Chapter 7

"There is a road from the eye to the heart that does not go through the intellect."—G. K. Chesterton

"...an organized live intelligent field is not exclusively exhibited by humans—it is the same live intelligent field observed in all forms of life."—Dr. G. Munger

Intelligent Live Information Field Expressions (LIFE) and Self-Healing

The current definition of "life" [1] does not incorporate the observation of a living field expression nor the presence and necessity of photons. (Note: the word life used in lower case letters refers to the current understanding of its definition. The word LIFE used in upper case letters creates an acronym meaning: intelligent Live Information Field Expression).

Both life and LIFE are observed as continuous cyclic events. I believe any definition of life that "terminates" or "ends" do not support this living cycle observation. Nor does it support a quantum continuum theory or a God concept understanding of this life cycle process. Quantum reality is not observed to create limits, promote annihilation, or incorporate dead ends. Human existence, which has contributed to and is inter-connected with all examples of life, provides logical, observable evidence to support a cyclic quantum continuum—a repeating circular expression of a LIFE continuum or God field expression continuum.

Nevertheless, **an organized intelligent live field is not exclusively exhibited by humans—it is the same live intelligent field observed in all forms of life.** Life is observed to be cyclic and never terminates—*it only transitions*. I believe a living expression, which is observed in all live organic life forms, is an information expression encoded or super-imposed on a photon, which originates from a universal Live Intelligent Information Field Expression and appears to be older than time.

Life was observed to exist on earth before humans and other advanced life forms appeared. In other words, "life" existed before humans (bacteria, plants, other animals etc.). This live observation equation is part of our biological reproduction cycle. For instance, a typical example of a life recycling in the human species is *partially* caused by the combining of male DNA and female DNA. However, a more complete understanding of this union would include the above-mentioned genomes combined with *environmental data intrusion* (such as toxins, disease, etc.) and non-material intrusions like *thought expressions (your RRT)*. Included in this would also be the constant flow of Photonic Information Expressions from a universal living information field—LIFE which directs and implements the combined DNA and other intrusions. This results in a modification of the DNA which eventually becomes a new version of a human.

Photonic Information Expressions can and do change your genetic blueprint (allowing an individual specific interpretation of physical and non-physical data). This is accomplished unconsciously by being constantly immersed in this living information field. However, by invoking an "intention to do so" we can, and do, alter our DNA with thought expressions. A new version, a species-specific re-creation of a human will emerge from this union which is a unique quantum biological entity—an individual-specific human expression. This "quantum expression" is independent, inter-connected and inter-dependent on the variables present in their DNA, their environment, and the information transmissions which are directions from LIFE itself (When I say "live DNA" I am saying the "living" aspect of this observation is ***separate*** from the DNA exhibited, and is actually Photon Information Expressions. DNA cannot achieve cell differentiation without the "live" factor being present). Nevertheless, this result may produce a new human that is stronger, healthier, and better adapted for their LIFE experience. Or just the opposite might happen, and a less than optimal birth would occur, perhaps even a still-born that would experience a death-transition.

This new life form (the infant) quickly learns its own way of evaluating environmental data **($K^r + P^r = MA$)**, which creates a modified sense of awareness. Previously it was mentioned that when your modified awareness is *repeated,* it creates a Reality Replication Template. Yes, even a baby is collapsing quantum waves of possibilities into particles of reality and creating its own version of its life experiences—this is wonderful beyond words; an intelligence which nurtures awareness and provides choice. Also previously mentioned is the Reality

Replication Template created by each of us that determines our current state of health and sets "your norm" or baseline perception of your health—homeostasis. Awareness of this process is the **key** to augmenting an innate self-healing awareness. Logically, you cannot utilize it if you do not know it exists. According to quantum physics, the power of "intension" collapses all possibilities you desire to experience into your reality—good or bad. It is you who makes this choice. I hope you will opt to choose your innate ability to augment this process.

As we grow, we automatically develop awareness using our version of the sensory data we collect from ourselves (egoic perception) and our environment(s). One way our specific health awareness can be observed is using a health observation guide, like the one utilized by [2] Dr. Paul Drouin of Quantum University. Dr. Drouin developed and assembled the "Seven Stages of Health" (Alarm, Adaptation, Exhaustion, Functional, Organic, and the Death. (However, for myself, I modified the 7th stage to include the word "transition" as I believe the current definition of death is incomplete). The Death-Transition experienced by a physical body exhibits a disconnection of its "living" field of Photon Information Expressions from its material manifestation (the physical body). This is not a termination or annihilation of these Photon Information Expressions—it is a transition for both the physical body and the "living" expressions we observe as a Life-force or intelligent organized animation. Let us explore this idea a little further.

The birth through death-transition is an observed Cycle of life; it is <u>not</u> observed to end with annihilation, nor is it observed to be created from nothing—it is cyclic. Life is derived from pre-existing life. The end of your physical life cycle is *transition*—not termination (Yep, you just keep going). Every material component of the human physical body is re-cycled, not destroyed. It eventually returns to gases, minerals and organic components and elements. (These components can be used over and over by other living organisms (cyclic) and are an example of a quantum continuation living-cycle process or a circular concept of LIFE). I believe a Photon Information Expression is an extension of a universal Intelligent Live Information Field Expression (LIFE) or, if you want to use the word God Expression, it will not disrupt the analogy or any of my equations. I believe all life form manifestations are part of LIFE. These field expressions are not subject to entropy, nor do they appear to be affected by the flow of time (NOTE: Do not confuse this with your live organic material expression of yourself—your physical body). These quantum field expressions leave the physical body because the body can no longer support, conduct, and/or maintain these Photon Information Expressions (your body is a living physical conductor, transmitter, and receiver. When a death-transition of the physical body occurs, the physical body becomes unable to conduct PIEs). In my opinion, once the physical body becomes denigrated to a point where it does not meet the minimum requirements to maintain and conduct these Photon Information Expressions, it experiences a death-transition. At this point, the Photon

Information Expression disconnects. Dang! A broken antenna.

A Photon Information Expression exhibits varying degrees of continuity or presence while interacting with a material living form. This continuity can be compared to the ability of a piece of copper wire to conduct electricity. For instance, the copper wire can be affected by corrosion, heat, cold, oxidation, breakage, etc. With these "varying degrees" of interference one can measure impaired electrical flow, and in the case of breakage, no flow of electrical current at all. (It is important to note that the source of electricity that flows through this piece of copper wire still exists, unless turned off, even if the wire is broken). A death-transition in the human body can be likened to the same type of "breakage" referred to in the broken copper wire example where the flow of electricity was interrupted. Like the copper wire, the Photon Information Expressions observed in a human body (or any living material form) can be impeded or disconnected (death-transition) but not annihilated—the living field expression *continues to exist*. However, it can no longer be received or transmitted from the physical body.

I believe a healthy physical body (animal, plant, fungus, etc.) continually receives and expresses these Photonic Information Expressions. This information provides all the components required for a physical body to remain functional. Current science believes life is exhibited by those that fit Dictionary.com's definition[3] and others, quoted below, "the condition that distinguishes organisms from inorganic objects and dead organisms, being manifested by growth through metabolism, reproduction, and the power of adaptation to environment through changes originating internally. The sum of the distinguishing phenomena of organisms, especially metabolism, growth, reproduction, and adaptation to environment. The animate existence or period of animate existence of an individual: to risk one's life; a short life and a merry one. a corresponding state, existence, or principle of existence conceived of as belonging to the soul: *eternal life*". Merriam-Webster [4] states 1: having life: not dead or inanimate. 2a: still in existence, force, or operation: active kept hope ***alive***. Merriam Webster (NOTE: These definitions are incomplete, and do not address a Photon Information Expression observation, nor do they address an "evolving" organism when the process appears to take millions of years, like some bacteria which express or some that refuse to evolve).

A physical death-transition is related to the interruption or disconnection of the LIFE's expressions (PIEs) from the physical body. However, some cells continue to function (they are still alive!) for a short time even when the interruption of the physical LIFE expression (a death-transition) causes the immediate interruption and transition of the PIEs governing the *overarching* species expression of an entity. **This is an observation that exhibits a single or multi-cellular expression as "alive", independent, interconnected, and inter-dependent with all its sub-systems and the**

over-all collection of cells which presents as a whole expression. This observation includes multiple live cellular expressions, or sub-systems, which when combined, comprise a group of cellular expressions like the lung, skin, heart, liver, etc. These multi-cellular expressions, or sub-systems, also exhibit a **"separate group awareness"** which is independent, interdependent, interconnected and directly supports the existence of a single species expression. A graphic, but crystal-clear example of this is severing the head from one's body. The logical conclusion is this physical body experiences a death-transition. From this observation, **we can conclude a single entity expression, i.e., a unicellular organism, exhibits a separate "life consciousness".** However, this individual's cell expression is also part of a sub-system (groups of cells, i.e., Liver, Heart, Lung, etc.) of a field of specific "live" cells which collectively create a sub-group consciousness. Additionally, these sub-systems create and support the existence of the whole awareness exhibited in a species. We can observe that the Photon Information Expressions are "intelligently" working together with these groupings of cells as independent and inter-dependent parts of a whole. A single cell expression of a life form exhibits the same Photon Information Expressions observed in each of the 37-40 trillion cells exhibited in the physical body of a human species. Live compartmental intelligence, inter-cooperation and organization are observed as present. This is an example of a live intelligent, organized field expression that manifests in a material form.

Let us expand on this concept. An observation of the physical human body is easily perceived as a "collective" comprised of single cells, multiple cells, and multiple groupings of cells, like your heart, lungs, bones, and organs. Additionally, Photon Information Expressions within these single or multiple groupings of cells (sub-systems) in humans and other species *are observed in each cell along with DNA.* You cannot combine the DNA of males with the dead ova of females and create live offspring. *This logically concludes a separate life force expression is present and necessary in biological reproduction.* I believe this cellular collective of information coordinates the retrieval of sensory data from your material and quantum environments. These examples of field expressions and consciousness are non-material concepts analyzed by the "mind" in conjunction with data recorded in the physical brain. This combination creates a Reality Replication Template—your understanding of this information and your perceived reality.

So, what is the experience of being "alive"? Once again, we get ambiguous definitions that appear incomplete. What we can logically extrapolate is it is <u>not</u> exclusively material. It is combined with Photon Information Expressions—a field observed to be manifested, conducted, stored and experienced by an organic living life form. Remember, the "live" field observation is *not* material. One can also observe that local environmental sensory data and non-local quantum data are contained and incorporated in this field expression (mind/body interaction which are independent and interdependent of each other). Photonic encoding of sensory data by the mind in conjunction with the brain exhibits a holographic collection of images and an encoding process (See Chapter 5, Photonic Encoding) which exhibits the existence of photonic information expressions as holographic images.

Just as a Photon Information Expression is a sub-system of LIFE, any "alive" expression can be observed as an inter-connected part of an operating system that uses Photon Information Expressions. The Photon Information Expression collects data from single or multiple groupings of live cell(s) for the purpose of promoting a *single entity awareness*—single cell or multi-trillion cells. These are intelligent and organized cellular manifestation(s) that share the same Photon Information Expressions. They create an overall or primary expression of a single species when interconnected. I believe this cannot be accomplished with any known technology or purely "reactive" responses between cells. This is due to the countless variables encountered in a live specie equation which can and do change constantly. This must be a live intelligent thinking response. Yes, I believe it is alive, aware, and part of you!

To re-iterate, it is important to note the Photon Information Expression is shown to collect and transmit varying degrees of intelligent awareness information which can be observed in a single cell as a stand-alone example of life or in a multi-cellular complex of intelligent groupings of cells (sub-systems) which create a complex and intricate *entire species specific expression.* This species-specific expression can contain multi-trillions of cells cooperating and coordinating their individual life expressions to "create" a live species-specific entity which appears to be more than the sum of its parts due to its quantum field interactions.

As discussed earlier, "death" is not an annihilation or termination. Anything that has life does not die; it only transitions its material and photonic field expressions into other observed forms (Yep! You do not die). The actual observation of a "life form" exhibits both material and non-material qualities likened to physical and field expressions. However, most humans give preference to the material aspects of this union. They utilize their physical senses in a manner that creates a priority for data that can be seen, touched, felt, etc. It appears most humans are not "aware" of the quantum observations—which are invisible, non-local and cannot be sensed using a material quantification methodology. Invisible is easy to overlook. (Ha!) Most of us need someone to point out these observations to us. If not, those that are unaware, omit them (a System of Interference) while creating their Reality Replication Template. This "omission" is due to the Photon Information Expressions being in the form of a non-material expression—which you cannot see or touch. As a result of this, human awareness personifies this life equation, imbuing it with human specific data conclusions (GRRTs) based on predominately *material observations* of data from their environment. This is a subjective conclusion created by our RRTs, LOLO effect, and Systems of Interference. A Group Reality Replication Template dominates the varying degrees of awareness in the human species. As mentioned above, material quantification is easier to understand because you can see it, touch it, feel it. Non-local data is "invisible" and not tangible. It requires awareness of its existence to actualize it. It requires *you* to utilize intent to know (An awareness aspect of your reality). However, being un-aware does not remove its vital importance to your RRT.

I believe the concepts of a Quantum Continuum, LIFE and God are essentially the same. Science and Spiritual concepts have dis-similar approaches toward understanding the life equation and all its complex states. It appears the thousands of years of "discussion" have blinded the human species' perceptions of science and spirit. This created GRRTs—Systems of Interference—a scotoma.

One of the problems associated with the word God is the ambiguity of linguistic determinism, semantics, and perceptions of the concepts and origins of the words associated with "God" and or "Gods". Also associated with this ambiguity is the confusion created when alternate definitions and understandings of the word "God" are used. For practical purposes I am stating in this chapter that God, a Quantum Continuum, the Infinite—no beginning and no end life concepts, are generally to be treated as the same. It is far too, too, too, exhausting to delve into the opinions from 196 countries,

50+ Bibles, 4,200, religions, 80,000 variations of these religions, interpreted by 7.7 billion people over a 5,000-7,000 year span (NOTE: If you wish to do a meta-analysis of these data, please send me a copy). However, the fact there are so many variations of religious concepts exhibits the complexity and ambiguity associated with interpreting these ideologies. The point to embrace here is *my intention* to bridge the philosophies of science, religion and spirit to produce a better understanding of the LIFE equation and create self-awareness and self-healing. It is NOT to promote one approach over the other, but rather, highlight the similarities inherent in these approaches toward a mutual understanding of this LIFE awareness analysis.

We have been learning about logical extrapolation and reasoning. I propose a question for your consideration: Is God, or a quantum continuum, aware that humans are not aware? This does not seem possible, due to the continual flow of LIFE's data to the TIC field expression which was mentioned previously. For instance: How hard would it be, hypothetically, for God or the other interpretations of a continuum, to prevent atrocities or pandemics? Why wouldn't they stop these unthinkable experiences? One explanation could be the **ignorance observed as part of human unawareness.** My observations are that most humans do not understand their participation in this equation. Is it possible that God, or the Quantum Continuum, allows this to happen because it is perceived to be what humanity desires? (What? Dang!) A sapient human live equation has the capability to collapse quantum waves of possibility into particles of reality just by "intending" to do so. Humans can collapse any reality into existence, so why do humans continue the insanity? The observation is *choice* NOTE: If you are not embracing self-awareness, this can be a bitter pill to swallow. My explanation infers that intervention is not experienced, because it is not required. The essence of "who you are", your individual specific interpretation, is not in danger (remember, you just transition; not die). We each can create an existence or reality that is free from the above-mentioned atrocities. Many do. You have a choice. Humans, as a species, has a choice—it is up to us as an individual person to change "our self" and to embrace scientific and spiritual enlightenment. By achieving this change of awareness, the human species is also affected. This happens one person at a time.

I concluded from the above discussion that the definition of "death" is incomplete.

Let us list some observations of a Photon Information Expression in a physical body:

Observation #1- We can observe a Live Intelligent Information Field Expression (LIFE) is cyclic and infinite.

Observation #2 -We can observe Photon Information Expressions are an extension of

LIFE and they radiate from a field and exhibit varying degrees of intelligent organizational qualities and awareness in various material cellular expressions as a live field.

a. Uni-cellular organisms

b. Multi-cellular organisms

c. Group specific sub-systems of cells within a larger multi-cellular organism

d. Like humans (Organs, bones, muscles, etc.)

e. An Individual material expression can be a specific multi-cellular organism

f. (Specie) and a Singular Quantum Intelligence (SQI) observed as an individual

g. Awareness in a material form

Observation #3-We can extrapolate that a Photon Information Expression is itself "alive". For instance, it can be observed that once the Photon Information Expression leaves or disconnects from the physical body, the physical body exhibits a death-transition. This logically concludes a ***live expression*** of some kind was previously there. I believe this field expression is a Photon Information Expression and that the Photon Information Expression is *alive*—it is a human observation experiencing something as alive. Once the Photon Information Expression is interrupted, a death-transition occurs and the physical body re-cycles back to basic elements. Additionally, all your sensory experiences, thoughts, images etc. are also observed to disconnect from the physical body at the same time the Photon Information Expression disconnects (the PIEs are carrying this data when the interruption occurs). This is a departure from the notion that life is solely an electro-bio-chemically based notion. It appears that a universal live intelligent organized field expression concept orchestrates and helps direct and maintain a live material manifestation.

Observation #4—A Photon Information Expression existed before any mammal manifestation experiences—before humans. LIFE existed prior to the appearance of a human interpretation of a life awareness. One would logically need a mind (non-local quantum event) and a brain (local material manifestation event) to perceive anything to be "alive", aware, or conscious as a human being.

Observation #5 – Life comes from life. All life forms are observed to come from something that is already alive (As of the date of this paper, no one has created life on our planet).

Observation #6 – DNA is a schematic or blueprint for biological replication which utilizes Photon Information Expressions. DNA requires instructions to assemble an individual specific life form. I believe it is the Photon Information Expressions, an extension of LIFE and epigenetic data retrieved from one's environments, both local and non-local, and directs this process.

Observation #7 – A Photon Information Expression is consistent with photonic observations being the prevalent data collection and transmission process of living experiences (pictures, images, thoughts—holograms). I believe data collected by Photon Information Expressions appear to be sub-atomic and are exhibited as photonic expressions (I believe all sensory information is super-imposed on photons—photonic encoding). Photons do not appear to be affected by the flow of time or entropy. Photons present as: particles, waves, or as transitions between these two states (We can logically hypothesize that photons are also data collectors).

Observation #8 – Photon Information Expressions can also be perceptions of knowledge (a thought) received from one's non-local environment (A quantum expression) and correlated with data from the physical brain. Both the local and non-local data is continually collected via our 19+ senses resulting in a modified awareness **($K^r + P^r = MA$).**

Observation #9 - A Photon Information Expression is observed as the live observation expression of a material manifestation (collector, conductor and emitter) and is observed as an extension of an infinite universal field accumulation of data I call an Intelligent Live Information Field Expressions-LIFE. Photon Information Expressions work in conjunction with both the individual specific material manifestation and with an "universal infinite original expression" to continue a live data collection process which is expressed as a circular continuum. I believe the Photon Information Expression directs and interprets schematics (DNA) and other unidentified environmental data for inclusion or exclusion in this endless cyclic of biological replication. A Photon Information Expression communicates with itself (it is a self-aware field--alive), the material body and the Live Intelligent Information Field Expression continuously. I hypothesize that this field expression is a quantifiable electromagnetic frequency, although I have not been able to isolate this frequency (yet!). It is this connection of the individual specific Photon Information Expression with the infinite database of a Live Intelligent Information Field Expression that facilitates communication between these expressions (and, as we are finding out, it is a two-way communication). As quantum beings we can tap into (the "knowing") and affect the Photon Information Expressions by using our ability to collapse quantum waves of possibility into particles of reality, using intention and observational feed-back.

This is relative to one's ability to perceive knowledge in the form of sensory data and subjectively interpret a desired outcome (intent). Each example of life and or species is, theoretically, becoming better and better each time the individual specific experiences of live male and female genomes are merged. However, the Reality Replication Template established by those unaware of this process can inhibit progress. It appears *your self-imposed limitations* and interpretation of environmental data take precedence over your genomic instructions and epigenetic data.

Observation #10 – Photon Information Expressions are included as part of the equation utilized in biological reproduction. Photon Information Expressions are the "life observation" or "alive" aspect associated with a genome. This means an "alive" ovum and an "alive" sperm form a zygote through a process referred to as cellular differentiation. This process is observed to initiate the following sequence of events: The Photon Information Expression instructs or orchestrates the DNA to replicate in a manner that includes local and non-local environmental data (epigenetic information interpretation). Through this process, the interpretation, the DNA, and other data are intelligently combined or implemented by Photon Information Expressions to create a new version of a species. Please remember, DNA are only blueprints or schematics. A separate intelligent living force (PIEs) orchestrates all the data both local and non-local to assemble and replicate a one of a kind species.

LIFE CYCLE

LIFE = a Live Intelligent Information Field Expression- > Photon Information Expression—as an extension of LIFE- > to DNA—a schematic or blueprint combined with environmental data both local and non-local, an epigenetic interpretation compiled and *interpreted* by an PIE to complete the reproduction of a live material manifestation. (Environmental data is included as epigenetic interpretation—both quantum intention and non-intended environmental intrusion can be included in this cycle: (**LIFE** > PIE> Birth > LIFE span > to Death-transition> **LIFE)**

Intelligent Living Information Field Expression

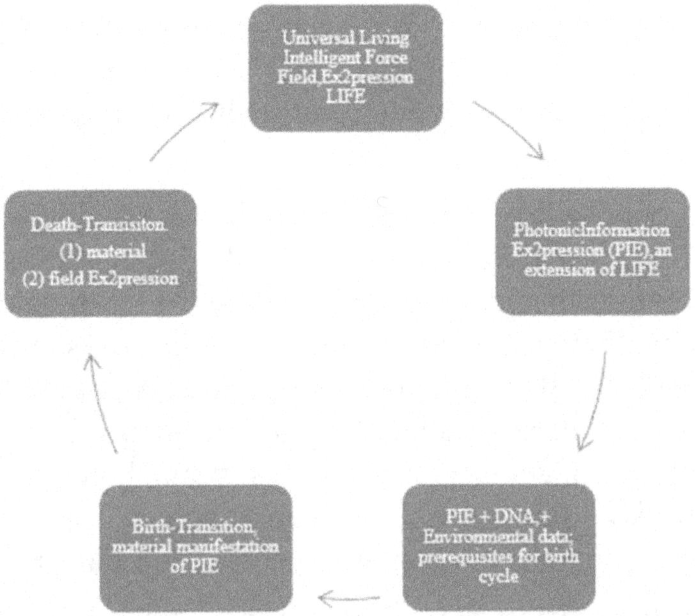

These instructions create a unique version of the merger of two (male and female) organisms. Photon Information Expressions are observed in a single cell, multi-cells, specific groupings of cells (intelligent sub-systems which exhibit intelligent organized quantifiable properties consistent with the observed material manifestations (brain, bones, skin, heart, liver, lungs, etc.). These sub-systems of intelligent groupings of cells are independent, interactive, and inter-dependent with all the other single cells, multi-cells, and sub-systems (the independent group-cell manifestations mentioned above) that comprise an over-arching representation of a species-specific organism. All group-cellular manifestations coordinate to re-create and maintain a complete species-specific organism. A common observation during this process is the sharing of species-specific DNA with every cell. This DNA equation is shared with, and located in, every single or multi-cellular grouping of cells.

I believe this observation requires a unifying intelligent field expression (PIE) which can interact, communicate and continually update the DNA contained within all independent and inter-dependent systems (37-40 trillion cells in humans) in a *fast as light manner*. This is a unicellular to multicellular to inter-dependent groupings of cells, as sub-systems (brain, bones, skin, heart, liver, lungs, etc.) which culminate in a species-specific organism or a single species "consciousness".

Observation #11 -- It is observed that all life forms (fields) exhibit movement, frequency, and the ability to conduct, store and interact with various other fields (Photons, electricity, electromagnetism, gravity, etc.). I believe these fields augment, diminish, have no effect, or create new fields when they interact. This collection creates inter-dependence with the individual specific interpretations of data collected from their environment.

The life equation consists of two (2ea) main classifications:

(1) A local material (physical body field collector) expression and

(2) A non-local Photon Information Expression, an extension of LIFE.

A material manifestation (physical body) completely recycles its material components upon experiencing a death-transition—if left alone to do so. The non-local Photon Information Expression components *cannot be destroyed*, they transition from one exhibited sub-expression (physical form) to another (a quantum field continuum form—LIFE). This live field does not change, it is just perceived to change due to the conduit or receptor (your body) being no longer functional. The data (stored as "thought" images) contained in these local and non-local fields are uploaded via our sensory experiences by Photon Information Expressions. It appears photons have an additional expression as a data collector and transmitter; Particle, Wave, Particle-wave, Wave-particle **and data collector and transmitter of information.** This assertion is based on data observed to exist in human off-spring which creates "instantaneous knowing" and the transfer of information not experienced in one's environment. For instance, child prodigies, idiot-savants and instant familiarity with mathematics, reincarnation, music prodigies etc. exhibit prior knowledge. I believe this literally means all information that has ever existed since the Big Bang, Big Bounce, Big Guess, or the God theory is *constantly* being recorded on images. I believe this data, which is imprinted on Photon Information Expressions, cannot be destroyed, and are collected and stored in an original infinite Live Intelligent Information Field Expression. This observation points us in the direction of the existence of a Live Intelligent Information Field

Expression. Nevertheless, this stored data provides a wonderful *continuity* for our life experiences and our consciousness of "all life" being independent, inter-dependent and inter-connected as part of the same original intelligent information field.

As mentioned previously, photonic images or holograms are stored in the human brain or neural like network of other living organisms. This is exhibited as an expression of photonic frequency and thus capable of transmission, reception, and measurement. Photonic images are experienced as sensory data in the here and now. They are also experienced as quantum thought expressions in your mind. Photonic images are experienced as dreams, thoughts, sight, etc. Photonic images are associated with organ transplant and memory(s) of a donor's transfer. For example, having a live organ transplant and instantaneously experiencing "new data" **not collected by you**. For instance, craving foods you never liked before, or experiencing data (images or pictures) you have never seen before. As was previously mentioned, the cells of a transplanted organ collect and share the same data as the whole organism. Why couldn't some of this "data" be transferred through the process of organ transplanting? Why do you think this information is observed in this manner?

Photons are collected by the human body and emitted in a seemingly chaotic manner. Photonic emissions are primarily concentrated in the head and shoulders regions of the human body [5]. Photons exhibit specific frequencies within the electromagnetic spectrum of radiation. Some of these visual frequencies have been documented to show access has been achieved by humans (See Remote Viewing examples provided by the U.S. CIA). [6] Additionally, near death-transition experiences are explained as photonic expressions. [7]

It is my belief that an infinite and complete data depository exists and is available to all those wishing or "intending" to access it. Give it a try! One practical way to tap into LIFE's collection of data is to observe (images) live organisms in nature with the *intention* of knowing something about them. This is a wonderful way to start!

If you are "searcher" or a "researcher" you will never be dissatisfied—rather, you will more likely be amazed at the already existing knowledge, engineering skills and intelligence the quantum aspect of Nature offers. This collection of data maybe older than this finite galaxy (and probably is), so remember not to limit your search to just the human experiences. If you utilize a cognitive observation you will be able to extrapolate data that displays logical conclusions—this will undoubtedly expand your awareness and establish a re-connection instantaneously. For example: Have you ever seen a spider's web in a bush or tree? Wouldn't this logically mean the spider observes (knows) insects fly? Why else suspend a webbed trap in the air and in a tree or bush to catch insects? Where did the spider learn to self-manufacture its web material? As previously mentioned, how does the spider know the spacing requirements or geometric designs for the web it spins?

How does the spider know how strong the web material should be? How long did it take to evolve a sac to store its web material in? Do you think the spider got help from an existing intelligent and organized quantum field expression? Or do you think it just happens? If you think it just happens, why? See where I am going with this line of inquiry? Always question observations—employ awareness.

How do some birds build their nests? Is it just a bunch of twigs and grasses? Or do they select specific building materials for warmth, drainage, anti-bacterial, anti-fungal and disease protection for their offspring? Many researchers believe it is an engineering marvel. [8] Where did they learn this?

You can utilize these types of observations to discover more about spiders and other LIFE forms in nature. This approach will expand your understanding of the entire expression of a spider or any other live organism. However, please remember to include *all* the data you are observing by using a systems integration approach—a combination of material and non-material observations—I believe this blending is the best approach.

What are your observations? How can you modify or replace this definition? Defining the Photon Information Expressions mentioned above will test your interactive, inter-connected self-awareness and create a thinking, feeling, loving, perplexing thought process which will move you toward self-awareness, self-confidence and consciousness. By comparing my definition and your definition with other definitions, you will gain more perception and knowledge. Note: Although a definition is important, remember the awareness one gains through analysis of the definition and its multiple possibilities is equally important. This awareness will guide your understanding of your individual specific reality of self-healing. It is OK to be wrong! Just keep gaining new awareness. Awareness plus intention can create consciousness (A + I = C) and develop your self-healing.

Definitions are an important part of this process.

Chapter 8

"We cannot discover ourselves without first discovering the universe, the earth, and the imperatives of our own being."—Thomas Berry

"...if you believe it, right or wrong, it affects your Reality Replication Template."—Dr. G. Munger

Problems with Definitions: Perceptions of Knowledge

When using your own innate ability to self-heal and gain awareness, *many* definitions can be problematic. If you believe something is true, you act on the information in a manner that supports your belief. This is accomplished by utilizing your individual specific Reality Replication Template, especially when the definitions are un-clear and ambiguous. Many times, definitions *allude* to an understanding, but fall short due to the nature of the data being defined. For instance, define intention, perception, love, or emotion. (See my partial list of definitions.) These and many other definitions require an individual specific interpretation of the *experience* created by these words (your Reality Replication Template) to understand it. This is a logical extrapolation using "your reasoning" combined with a cognitive understanding of your language. However, this can also be defined as a "stab" or "guess" based on interpretation. This approach inserts Systems of Interference in an etymological definition process which skew data—be careful.

What is the definition of the word definition? Is this definition clear? Contained in the definition below, where does it state the accuracy of the statement? It gives a generalized subjective interpretation that leaves you unsure of what is being stated. For example, Merriam-Webster's definition can be defined [1] as: "**1a:** a statement of the meaning of a word or word group or a sign or symbol dictionary *definitions* **b:** a statement expressing the essential nature of something **c:** a product of defining **2:** the action or process of stating the meaning of a word or word group **3a:** the action or the power of describing, explaining, or making definite and clear the *definition* of a telescopeher comic genius is beyond *definition* **b (1):** clarity of visual presentation **:** distinctness of outline or detail improve the *definition* of an image **(2):** clarity especially of musical sound in reproduction **c:** sharp demarcation of outlines or limits a jacket with distinct waist *definition.*"

See what I mean? This definition, if used by you, would be considered a System of Interference because it does not say anything; it only alludes to an understanding. Would not images of information be better? So, you make your own definition based on what you "think" it means. It alludes to an individual specific interpretation of a definition but misses the mark. Perhaps a better definition should be coined and re-coined until a more exacting interpretation can be logically agreed upon by as many people as possible—a GRRT of definitions. What do you think? The point is, it is non-descript and therefore misleading and incomplete. **Nevertheless, you use it as a fact-based definition!**

During my investigation of word meanings, it was easier to define a physical "something" using a material methodology than it was a non-material "something" using a material methodology. Physical measurement utilizes varying degrees of reductionistic science observations using your individual specific interpretation of agreed upon sensory data definitions (physical properties, height, weight, length, color, etc.). The ambiguity with "definitions" becomes more acute when qualitative, cognitive, non-local experiences are inserted into a quantitative methodology model. This leaves the "definition" incomplete and skewed. You cannot add 3 apples and 3 oranges and get 6 apples. Nor can you exclude the oranges because they can't equate in the apple equation (This is an example of Systems of Interference; excluding data). What is required is an integrative methodology which combines two or more "measuring sticks" so to speak, to measure and compile ALL the data observed to be present in the analysis (oranges and apples).

Many definitions defy definition using a measuring type methodology (intention, perception, knowledge, and countless more). How can you get an ounce of intention or a foot of intention? What color is knowledge? How heavy is perception? Instead, the definition is ambiguous, and for all intents and purposes, unusable as an accurate metric. Nevertheless, many non-material experiences humans observe, and experience are agreed upon as "real"—just not definable using a measuring type methodology. This makes the understanding even more difficult (your Reality Replication Template becomes combined with ambiguous definitions, oops!). So, how do we define non-material/non-physical experiences? We can use a qualitative methodology and logical extrapolation. In other words, we use our perception of the observation to make a logical interpretation of what is experienced. Then we share our data with others and see if the logic is sound. This is contingent on our Reality Replication Templates, Lock-on Lock-out effect, Systems of Interference, and our self-awareness. For instance, if we use the bumble bee orchid as an example, we can state the following: The bumble bee orchid morphs part of its labellum to resemble a female bumble bee. From this you can logically extrapolate the bumble bee orchard can detect visible light-waves (it can see) and creates this 3D photonic image of a female bumble bee. The logic being: How can it sculpt an image if it cannot (see) detect it? Not only that, but the male bumble bee is fooled by it also. Many observations defy a material measuring type definition and cannot be understood with this approach. Other definitions were taught in school as though they were factual. For instance, the internet provides hundreds of examples of what a generalized example of an atom is supposed to look like. It is taught in physics classes. [2] It is a circle representing an atom, with other dots representing electrons orbiting around this atom. However, until the year 2018, no one had ever photographed an atom. As remarkable as I think this photo is, it is still just a dot [3] (go to this website and see for yourself). Do you see any electrons rotating around the "dot"?

CAUTION: Definitions that are un-questioned and *not factual* still support the reality you experience as your Reality Replication Template (**if you believe it, right or wrong, it affects your Reality Replication Template**). Definitions should be continually scrutinized to include the most reasonable extrapolations and latest discoveries. This awareness requires vigilance on your part to keep you abreast of these Systems of Interference and their effect on your ability to comprehend definitions. Remember, any definition, **if believed**, affects your awareness and RRT**.** Consequently, this awareness affects your ability to self-heal.

How do definitions affect self-healing? If you believe something is true, it is (at least to you). However, this does not mean it is necessarily factual. Science consistently exhibits data they believe is factual, and they have even taught it to others (me included). For instance, in the 15th century, the best universities in the world believed the planet was flat. In the 17th century, scholars believed the earth's star (our Sun) revolved around the earth. Medical science in the 17th century did not believe in "invisible" things call germs. In the 18th century, doctors and others believed mercury (please exclude homeopathic dilutions) could be given to patients as a cure. The list goes on and on. What we once <u>thought</u> of as correct gets superseded by new discoveries (I believe this is a good thing! Welcome to scientific investigation).

However, we should constantly emphasize that our track record proves factual data is temporary, at best. Our goal should be to continuously expand scientific awareness within ourselves and medicine, and in the investigative methods we utilize.

So, how does all of this affect your ability to self-heal?

With the advance of quantum medicine, we are finding "your thoughts" are much more important than ever before. As previously mentioned, your thoughts (especially intentions) create and shape your reality. The mind/body connection is an observable experience and qualitatively definable (See Chapter 19, Mind-Body Interactions). How you think a creative expression is exhibited in your physical, vital, mental, supra-mental, and quantum bodies? [4] (Thank you Quantum University). These thought expressions determine your self-healing awareness.

Due to this expanded awareness, it is important to collect as much data about yourself as possible. Get to know your body and mind and the expressions (specific to you) that are indicators of your "individual" state of health. This is always a good beginning! Change your Reality Replication Template so you are willing to experience a quantum leap of understanding with respect to your definition and the experience of self-healing—"intend" to change.

Humans are content with approximations or generalized information (See Chapter 15, Subjective

Memory Experiment). The problem with this is we don't acknowledge the problems inherent in this evaluation (Lock-on Lock-out effect, Systems of Interference and Reality Replication Templates). As previously mentioned, humans evaluate definitions to fit their own Reality Replication Template. Definitions affect your individual specific perception and knowledge. This fact makes it imperative to be continually aware of the Lock-on Lock-out Effect and Systems of Integration that directly affect your Reality Replication Template. Without intending this, you can remain in a mental state referred to as invincible ignorance that is related to the unaware version of your RRT. This mental block inhibits or prevents your ability to access new data! This is a negative experience of being stuck in a Reality Replication Template (no awareness of your RRT) and is not conducive to your overall health.

It is uncomfortably common to hear people state a theory or hypothesis as a fact! Here is one example. When I ask students the question, "How did the universe come into being?" the response is, "Big Bang" or "Big Bounce"—which are **only theories**. Or, they say God built it. But, once again, there is no way of knowing. NOTE: It is not the purpose of this chapter to debate any of the above-mentioned theories. Its purpose is to illustrate Reality Replication Templates and individual specific interpretation of data which has not been confirmed.

<u>BEWARE OF DEFINITIONS!</u> They can impair <u>your</u> quantum signature of self.

In our quest to become more aware of our ability to self-heal, we have been discussing new awareness and perceptions of knowledge. Some of these perceptions avoid definitions which would include other animals and or plants. We are taught that the Plant Kingdom and the Animal Kingdom are separate and have no connection. This is not the observation (i.e. yarsagumba, in Nepal, half plant, half animal.). Nevertheless, any inclusion of sentience and sapience with plants is rejected by most of the scientific community. In fact, rigid separatism is so apparent that is screams anthropomorphism when interpreted by humans. Anthropomorphism promotes the idea that humans are "more than" other life forms and are the exclusive recipients of sapience. This is not observed to be factual (see definition of Quantum Phyto-Sapience).

Let us look at a few uncomfortable "human" definitions which affect *your* reality.

"Kill [4] is to deprive of life**:** cause the death of, a disease that has *killed* thousands He threatened to *kill* them. **b(1):** to slaughter (an animal) for food **(2):** to convert a food animal into (a kind of meat) by slaughtering **2a:** to put an end to *kill* competition a change that could *kill* our chances for success **b:** DEFEAT, VETO *killed* the amendment **c:** to mark for omission *also* **:** DELETE *kill* a quote**d:** ANNIHILATE, DESTROY *kill* an enemy."

Humans must kill to stay alive. (What?) Whether you kill plants or animals, you are required to interrupt their Photon Information Expressions and force the transition of their physical manifestation back into basic elements. You are a killer. (Do not confuse this with a murderer; although I believe randomly killing plants for no purpose is a form of murder or forced transition!) How does this definition resonate with you? Do you feel like you are doing anything wrong? When you read this definition, what emotions are stimulated? If a grizzly bear (or other carnivore) killed a human for food, would you perceive this as wrong? What would you think if a human killed another human for food? What emotions are you experiencing reading this? Do you exalt yourself and believe this does not apply to you? Why is this observed to be the "LIFE Equation" exhibited by Nature to sustain life on earth? "From life comes life." Does the definition fit the observation? Should we change it? Do you think we are missing part of the picture here? Awareness needs to be applied to this definition! What do you think?

Although photosynthesis can sustain some plants indefinitely—many plants **opt** to kill animals to supplement their specific nutritional needs. Why do plants kill animals to stay alive? There are 750+ carnivore plants listed online. [5] Humanity needs to redefine the word "Kill"—it is not what we observe, and it's not what we "think". How old is this definition? It appears that ancient linguistic determinism may have played a factor in the writing of this definition, a definition that was never updated. The definition of the word "kill" requires a more comprehensive understanding to be incorporated. (Send me an example of what you believe.)

To reiterate, killing something automatically insists it is alive. However, as previously mentioned, it does not terminate or annihilate it, but rather "transitions" the material expression of this life form (recycles its physical form back to basic elements) and interrupts the Photon Information Expressions creating a Death-Transition. To kill something, creating a death-transition so it is no longer in existence, is not observed. Therefore, this definition of kill is not a logical assumption or a reasonable definition. Termination does not support a quantum cyclic existence. How do you kill (destroy or annihilate) the observable non-material "Photon Information Expression" in any species? How do you kill an information field? How about a frequency in the electromagnetic spectrum of radiation—a light expression? A "Photon Information Expression" or "life force observation" is a non-local observation which is not material and contains no physical components—it cannot be "killed". I believe the definition of life's cycle should not be a fear based, emotionally terminating experience.

The word "kills", as it pertains to living organisms, is observed as a combination of material and non-material transitions--not annihilation. This ideology promotes a cycle of continuation, a feed-back loop or circular experience. A Photon Information Expression must be an Expression of a quantum circular continuum to fit the definition proposed in quantum mechanics—no beginning and no end. It is cyclic and originates from a Live Intelligent Information Field Expression.

Please remember, a Photon Information Expression is combined with a birth through death-transition cycle of life. Your life cycle is transitional, not terminal. In other words, the physical body can no longer receive or transmit data. The definition of "kill" could use some updating. What do you think?

This leads us to the definition of death.

Neither God, nor a quantum continuum, exhibit any evidence that material items are taken with you when you experience a death-transition. I agree with this observation—you do not take anything tangible with you when you experience a death-transition. If you believe in God (choose any of the 4,200 religions and/or 80,000 variations used in 196 countries over the last 5,000 years), the observation is the same. You only take your Photon Information Expressions, encoded with memories of images of your life experiences on earth. These images are recorded in a database in a LIFE continuum as a single entity awareness—*you*. Death-transition is the separation of the "Photon Information Expressions" which are experienced as intelligent and organized conscious field expressions collecting and transmitting data from a material body (animal, plant, fungus, etc.). This body must express and emit a live field expression to be considered alive. However, according to this definition, life is experienced as [6] being "...organisms are open systems that maintain homeostasis, are composed of cells, have a life cycle, undergo metabolism, can grow, adapt to their environment, respond to stimuli, reproduce and evolve. 1: having life: not dead or inanimate. 2a: still in existence, force, or operation: active kept hope *alive*. Merriam Webster." (These definitions are observations of a physical form and do not include any quantum field expressions. This means this current definition of the word "death" is incomplete).

What attracts and maintains this "Photon Information Expression" while manifested in physical form? Do live cells play a role? Can varying degrees of health affect the observed status of a Photon Information Expression? The observation is yes! A **live** physical manifestation, you, acts like an antenna or collector for the LIFE force expression. Does the health or maintenance of your body affect healing? Once again, the logical conclusion is yes. The mind affects the body and the body affects the mind—your awareness interpretation of your RRT. If the physical body, as a collector, is damaged, diseased, impeded or altered, it affects reception and transmission of the Photonic Information Expressions. This infers that self-healing is concerned with the maintenance of the physical body. The physical body requires this transmission and reception of live field expressions to stay alive and healthy.

The death-transition recycles the physical form back to its basic components and the non-local Photon Information Expression is transferred back to the Living

Intelligent Information Field Expression (LIFE). However, this is not an all or nothing event. Remember, some cells continue living even when the death-transition has occurred. For example: Blood, lymph, sera can live 15 – 35 minutes after your head is removed from your body. **This means that "alive" is a Photon Information Expression" and it is present in the individual sub-system(s) of life as a single cell or multi-cell expression**. The physical body experience is a collective of multiple single and multi-cellular Photon Information Expressions. Each of the 37-40 Trillion cells in the human body exhibits a Photon Information Expression and DNA. I cannot say this enough. It is this collection of information (quantum data) that creates our non-local sense of "awareness and consciousness". This awareness is experienced by the "mind" and shared with the physical brain for recordation in accordance to how we created our Reality Replication Template. I believe this field expression is alive.

So, what is the experience of being "alive"? Once again, we get ambiguous definitions from current science. What we can extrapolate is that it is <u>not</u> material. It is almost always exhibited or manifested in organic material forms. **This logically concludes that being "alive" is a quantum field expression, not a material construct.**

Does a field (Electromagnetic, Gravitational, etc.,) continue to exist after the destruction of the physical presence expressing it is removed? Of course! I also believe data collected by Photon Information

Expressions are transmitted and contained in the original Live Intelligent Information Field Expression—a photonic information field continuum which does not disintegrate. I believe this data is "you" specific, but also continues to be part of the Live Intelligent Information Field Expression integrated as part of the whole. I believe this is photonic encoding of sensory data by the mind to the brain. This process exhibits a holographic or image collection of your data that is not affected by the flow of time (See Chapter 5, on Photonic Encoding).

There is both an intelligence and an organizing principle associated with Photon Information Expressions. LIFE itself is organized in a manner that perpetuates this expression—and it continues indefinitely. This intelligent organizing principle constantly provides subjective examples of awareness expressions or Reality Replication Templates.

This means the current definition of "death" is incomplete and should be expanded.

1. The material body re-cycles back to basic elements.

2. A Photon Information Expression disconnects un-altered from the material body; and does not terminate, but rather is transmitted back to this existing field -- LIFE.

3. A Photon Information Expression becomes part of the human data collective field experience or the Total Information Continuum, a "universal quantum memory" of all live data experiences.

4. A Photon Information Expression is part of a quantum field continuum or God concept.

Is a quantum concept of the mind alive/aware/conscious? Does the mind work in conjunction with all other "live" physical manifestation of sub-systems (Cells, organs, bones, environment etc.)? I believe yes. The "mind" and brain are bridged or inter-connected to one another. A connection which allows neurogenesis to occur via the thought expression of "intention". *This bridging is a non-material experience which causes a physical manifestation!* This is not something from nothing, but rather a physical expression created from an existing quantum field. Nevertheless, this "bridge" between your brain and mind is where your concept of kill, death, life, and every other awareness perception exists. Yes, you create this. This is your belief or individual specific variation of this data.

Other definitions referred to in human history are incomplete and bias. Just because you quote a reference does not make it valid. It is always good to re-think and, if necessary, revise most definitions. If your observation is readily exhibited, analyze it to see if the definition fits the observation.

Remember, your individual quantum experience does not terminate upon death-transition. Neither a quantum theory nor a God theory prescribes to this belief.

The above analysis delineates the problems inherent in definitions. Luckily, our next chapter examines plants, their intelligence, and how they support our health and our very existence. I believe we should all be grateful for LIFE's intelligent, organized, and balanced equation of existence. Part of this "balanced equation" is the contribution plants provide—without plants, most, or all, species on earth would perish.

Chapter 9

"This logic also includes any living organism that satisfies these same requirements for being intelligent, sentient, or sapient—like those exhibited by plants."
—Dr. G. Munger

Live Plants Support Self-Healing?

Without plants, humans would perish. Plants feed and clothe us, create a breathable atmosphere, and much more. In addition to this, plants have provided a viable source of medicine since our beginnings here on earth. Plants support human existence and provide healing properties to help your body mitigate and cure disease. New research on diet, nutrition, and health awareness is expanding this observation and reaffirming the inter-connectedness we once commonly embraced together.

Many plants exhibit signs of intelligence. However, the word "intelligence" is still, for the most part, considered a human attribute despite evidence to the contrary. According to Merriam-Webster [1], the word intelligence is defined as, "the ability to learn or understand or to deal with new or trying situations." Plants are continually learning, understanding, and dealing with trying situations such as deforestation, toxic dumping, humans, GMO, climate alteration and more. Many plants fit the following definition of intelligence (See Chapter 10, Bumble Bee Orchid).

The intelligence which occurs in plants does so as varying degrees of phyto-sentience and phyto-sapience. This is a plant's ability to experience an awareness of their environment and their selves. Many plants exhibit the ability to think and reason and have the capacity to recall information.

Researchers studying plant intelligence have yet to agree upon a definition of this attribute, so I submit the above expanded definition using the following equations. **(rSd + MA + Res = SA)** = Memory (recorded sensory data) + Modified awareness + reasoning = Sapience and **(A +P + rSd + SI + SAP = SR)** ergo Awareness + perception + memory + systems of interference + Sapience = a subjective reality (modified awareness or RRT).

These equations exhibit the presence of intelligence in many plants. However, it is important to note this *is not an all or nothing concept*. Human beings <u>also</u> exhibit varying degrees or percentages of intelligence. These degrees or percentages are experienced by all humans regardless of their education. Some humans show a higher degree of cognitive understanding and can comprehend data which is more complex and sophisticated than other humans. [2] Humans have devised many different methods to test the intelligent quotient (IQ) of humans. This can range from 70 to 145+ (a significant difference or range, degree or percentiles depending on whose methods you employ to quantify this data). Most of us grew up with an alpha-numeric system for evaluating intelligence in school, either letter grades like A, B, C, D, F, or a percentage range from 0 to 100 that graded performance. Although antiquated, this type of intelligence quantification indicates an observable difference. How can we determine if a plant is sentient and or sapient when defined in a general conceptual linguistic context? Determining plant intelligence requires observations and logical reasoning. One is required to compile as much material data as you can and analyze this data using a quantitative methodology. Then you need to compile as many non-material observations as you can utilizing a qualitative methodology. Now, combine these data and methodologies and prepare to be astonished!

While all humans are sentient, not all humans are sapient. Brain damaged humans, mongoloid idiots, idiot-savants and the mentally impaired, do not possess all the requirements to be considered *a full member* of this group's classification. However, as stated above, varying degrees of sapience have been established using "words" which indicate examples of being less-than. Ergo, if a human meets the minimum requirements of this definition—they are considered intelligent or sapient. **This logic also includes any living organism that satisfies the same requirements for being intelligent, sentient, or sapient—like those exhibited by plants**. I chose a specific example to illustrate this—the bumble bee orchid, Ophrys-Bombyliflora (This will be elaborated on in Chapter 10, Bumble Bee Orchid).

Human beings exhibit the largest percentage of sapience. This is readily evident in their accumulation of data (millions of books, video recordings and the analyzation of that data). No other species does this. However, sapience is individual specie specific by varying degree. Asserting that sapience is a trait recognized only in human beings is an antiquated anthropomorphic construct. This assumption injects Systems of Interference into the analysis and rejects viable evidence to the contrary. In conjunction with my observations of the bumble bee orchid, I screened for Systems of Interference and came to the logical conclusion: *the bumble bee orchid is both sentient and sapient.*

Examples of Plant Intelligence

According to Stefano Mancuso [3], et.al, "a plant's functions are not related to organs, which means plants breathe without lungs, nourish themselves without a mouth or stomach, and stand erect without a skeleton." Plants do not have a spleen, liver, pancreas, or heart. Nor do they have a brain (cerebral cortex) like humans. Organs are not present in plants because they are **not required**. Correlating plant data to fit animal data (organs, and especially the human brain) is not rational and confers bias. Plants and animals are classified into different scientific kingdoms, and a massive amount of data clearly delineates the differences between the Plant Kingdom and Animal Kingdom. **As you will learn in this chapter, plants do not need eyes to see, ears to hear, or a brain to experience their environment.**

Determining intelligence is a cognitive evaluation based on definitions, observations, and scientific methodology. As a researcher, it becomes problematic since I am an animal (human) in the process of examining and analyzing plants. I am pre-disposed to Systems of Interference and diploma mill indoctrination of what the scientific community considers factual and acceptable evidence. An incredulous version of plant intelligence to avoid is that of Mr. Potato Head, a toy that children played with years ago in which they attached various plastic parts (eyes, nose, arms, legs, feet, hat, etc.) which resembled human appendages and apparel, to potatoes or other types of vegetables. This is a comical example of anthropomorphism—a bias Reality Replication Template. However, many still cling to this basic construct which requires plants to be *human-like* if they are to be considered intelligent.

My awareness of these pre-existing Systems of Interference act as a system of "checks and balances" providing constant feed-back during the empirical observation process. **Scientific evidence of any kind should never be omitted; systems of interference of any kind should never be included**. The following examples of plants will exhibit various observations of intelligent plant responses and a logical extrapolation of cognitive meanings which are associated with the plant kingdom and plant intelligence.

1. Tobacco Plant: According to the Max-Planck Institute in Jena, Germany [4], wild tobacco plants emit volatile organic compounds (VOCs) when a hawkmoth

larva attacks the tobacco plant. A VOC is emitted into the air and calls other insects that prey on the hawk moth larva thus employing a defense strategy to insure survival.

This exhibits an understanding of the hawkmoth larva and of the other insects that are called upon for help. How does the tobacco plant "*know*" that a larva's specific VOC will call an insect to rid them of this pest? This quantification still eludes researchers. However, if they use a qualitative methodology, the evidence suggests that the tobacco plant knows. *Nevertheless, the VOC exists; demonstrating the tobacco plant's ability to perform this function*. Logic concludes the tobacco plant is aware of this data and *remembers* to utilize it when needed. As previously mentioned, the tobacco plant also demonstrates the ability to manufacture a hawkmoth larva specific pheromone (VOC). Where did it get the formula to create the VOC? Was this from a direct contact with the hawkmoth? Logically, one can examine the material manifestation, the VOC, and acknowledge it exists. The fact that it physically exists, demonstrates that the tobacco plant has an awareness of its environment, the hawkmoth larva, enemies of the hawkmoth larva, reproductive habits, and intelligent design.

(2) Corn Plant: Corn plants also use VOC or pheromones [5] to call parasitic wasps that kill worms attacking the corn plant and lay their eggs inside these worms.

This demonstrates the corn plant's awareness of parasitic wasps and the corn plant's observation that the wasps lay their eggs inside these worms. This exhibits an understanding of the reproductive habits of the parasitic wasps and demonstrates the ability of the corn plant to manufacture VOCs.

(3) Tomato Plant: The tomato plant not only emits pheromones to call the horned worm wasp [6] to attack and lay their eggs in the hornworm, they also exhibit the ability *to hear sound vibrations.* When researchers recorded the sound of a hornworm eating the leaves of a tomato plant and played back the recording in the presence of the tomato plant at a later time (memory), the tomato plant responded defensively as though it was actually being eaten in that moment by a hornworm. Consequently, the tomato plant emitted an alarm pheromone to call the horned worm wasp.

This shows the ability of the tomato plant to hear sound vibrations, remember the sound of their leaves being gnawed off and to synthesize a chemical defense (VOC).

(4) Mimosa Pudica can be taught, and it remembers. The mimosa pudica is a plant that reacts to touch. If you touch its leaves they close and the stems droop. Monica Gagliano, a research ecologist at the University of Western Australia in Perth, experimented [7] with the mimosa pudica by dropping the plant in a manner (her words) "similar to an amusement park thrill ride." This was comprised of 7 sets of 60 drops each in a one-day

period. During the drops, the mimosa pudica's leaves shut tight. However, the mimosa pudica quickly **learned** not to react at all. Dr. Gagliano waited three days and tested them again. Still no reaction. She went back 6 days later and repeated this experiment. The plant had learned not to react to the dropping exhibited in the experiment. In addition to the mimosa pudica exhibiting memory, it exhibits the act of closing its leaves and drooping when touched. This is an example of the mimosa pudica demonstrating a sense of feeling.

(5) Acacia trees, according to Wouter Van Hoven, zoologist from Petroia University, "produce tannin in quantities lethal to the Kudu antelope that eat their leaves." [8] Additionally, an alarm signal or pheromone is emitted into the atmosphere to warn other acacia trees of the danger. This is accomplished by the acacia tree emitting ethylene into the air that can travel up to 50 yards. Van Hoven is quoted to say, "…this happens within 5 to 10 minutes of the tree experiencing or realizing it is being eaten. The Acacia (Acacia drepanolobium) has also developed a symbiotic relationship with an aggressive biting ant (Crematogaster) that lives on the Acacia, makes their nests, and eats the sweet nectar provided by the acacia. In return, these ants swarm when invaders, like the antelope, start eating the plant." [8]

This undoubtedly shows awareness of one's environment and the ability to synthesize tannin which is used as a defense against the Kudu antelope. It also shows the ability to synthesize ethylene (pheromone) to warn other acacia trees of the impending survival danger (a sense of community). The acacia tree has developed a relationship with the crematogaster ant showing awareness of the ant and its dietary requirements. These are thoughtful and reasonable responses to impending dangers. These acts exhibit intelligent expression—thought.

(6) According to Newitz and Karpinski, [9] "Plants can remember the light they have experienced" (memory). Also, according to Anna PIE Newitz, and Dr. Professor Stanislaw Karpinski, "Plants are able to assess their environment by analyzing light and are able to "remember" light they have experienced recently. By analyzing chemical reactions in leaves, scientists have come to appreciate that plants possess a kind of intelligence."

(7) According to Dr. Alex Webb, lead researcher at the University of Cambridge, [10] The Arabidopsis Thaliana plant can tell time. Dr. Webb is also quoted as saying, "Inhibiting photosynthesis, for example, slowed the plants internal clock by between 2 and 3 hours. This exhibits an ability to calculate time intervals."

These are just a few examples of plant intelligence. A quick perusal of the internet will result in locating many professional journals and scientific articles expounding on the amazing discoveries in the field of plant intelligence.

Wikipedia's definition [11] for plant intelligence is ambiguous. Wikipedia alludes to perception as the mechanism to understand intelligence. This required me to coin my own definition: *Plant intelligence is varying degrees of sapience which are exhibited by a plant's ability to be aware of its environment, be aware of themselves, think, reason, and exhibit the capacity for memory.*

Plants re-act and interact within their environments. Plants communicate with each other and with other species, using alarm pheromones, photons, underground interaction of root systems and most of the same senses that humans use, including hearing, feeling, touch, seeing, proprioception, tasting, thermoception, and many more (See the sensory chart in Chapter 1). Plants have learned to solve problems within their local ecosystem in a manner which seldom harms it. This includes quantum biological awareness and the *plant's ability to collapse quantum waves of possibility into local reality*. This observation was not previously identified or attributed to the plant kingdom. It is now an observation noted in this chapter.

According to Science Daily, [12] "some plants (cycads) heat up and emit an odor that makes the male pollen covered insects leave the cone and then use a milder odor to attract the insects into female cones, thus facilitating fertilization." The bumble bee orchid uses "sexual deception" to cause male bumble bees to be attracted to its flower by producing a virgin female bumble bee sex pheromone which is emitted into the air; combining this with a visual 3-dimensional representation which resembles a female bumble bee. [13]

"These deceptions cause the males to attempt to copulate (false copulation) with the orchid labellum." [14] During this process pollen becomes attached to the males and is then taken to other flowers helping with pollination.

Orleans states, [15] "Other species of orchids imitate the shape of a specific insect which the pollinating insect likes to kill; called pseudo-antagonism." This indicates an intricate understanding of the insects' social culture and environment. During the attack, the insect becomes covered with pollen and then takes this pollen to the next plant where the insect repeats this same mistake thus aiding in the fertilization process. Are specific plants intentionally engineering their appearance to attract a specific insect? The hammer orchid and its hinged bucket design are quite remarkable. The male hammer wasp detects the pheromone of the female wasp, which does not fly, and the male flies toward the source of the scent (pheromone) only to find a replica of the female hammer wasp. Normally, what happens is the male wasp picks up the female and flies away, copulating with her in the process. However, the hammer orchid has not only fooled the male wasp with a pheromone and a 3-D replica of the female wasp, but has engineered a hinging mechanism that is capable of dumping the male wasp over and over into the hammer orchids pollen as it repeatedly tries to fly away with the decoy. [16] This indicates the ability to see and experience its environment and to create a complex strategy to lure the male bee to its flower. It also exhibits an understanding of engineering of how to make and utilize a hinge to insure saturation of pollen on the male bee during this deception.

These examples undoubtedly display a knowledge and awareness of their environment. The hammer orchid exhibits the ability to select a specifically chosen insect. It understands the selected insect's mating habits. Like the bumble bee orchid, the hammer orchid displays knowledge of chemistry and engineering.

Plant Awareness

A new definition of plant awareness is required to understand the relationships plants have with their environment. Recent research has proven that plants are no longer thought of as just reactive in their environment, but rather interactive (See Examples of Plant Intelligence above). This observation is true about the bumble bee orchid as well. A new definition must include the plant's ability to interact with specific and complex aspects of their environment and exhibit the logic of conscious choice or intent if they exhibit it. Current research in this area logically includes cognitive and quantum aspects of understanding with a conclusion that some plants are sentient and others sapient. According to Stefano Mancuso [18] et.al, plants constantly monitor their environment and, in the process, utilize 20 senses (See Chapter 1, Sensory Data of Plants and Animals).

Relative to this discussion is my plant awareness survey I conducted (See below). The diploma mill indoctrination which exists regarding this subject is no longer viable. However, it is interesting to note the results of this small survey which indicate a slight resistance to calling plants intelligent. This is true even when data is provided which states a fact, "If a plant emits an alarm pheromone that calls an insect to its aid, do you think the plant knows this specific insect exists (See question #1)? In conjunction with Quantum University, I was able to circulate a "Plant Awareness Survey" via Survey Monkey, to test the general awareness of this group of people about plant intelligence. This survey indicates a sampling of what this population's awareness is regarding plant intelligence. The results are as follows:

Plant Awareness Survey Results

Question (1)

If a plant emits an alarm pheromone that calls an insect to its aid, do you think the plant knows this specific insect exists?

Total respondents = 75

60 responds answered Yes = 80 %

15 responds answered No = 20 %

Question (2)

Is it logical to extrapolate that if a plant knows one insect in its environment that it knows others?

Total respondents = 74

1 respondent skipped.

65 respondents answered Yes = 87.84 %

9 respondents answered No = 12.16 %

Question (3)

A tomato worm is eating a tomato plant. The tomato plant emits an alarm pheromone to attract the horned worm wasp which kills the tomato worm and lays its eggs in it. Do you think the tomato plant knows this when it is calling the horned worm wasp for help?

Total respondents = 75

57 responds answered Yes 76 %

18 responds answered No = 18 %

Question (4)

Do you think the tomato plant knows it is attracting the horned worm wasp?

Total respondents = 75

55 respondents answered Yes = 73.33 %

20 respondents answered No = 26.67 %

Question (5)

It has been proven that the bumble bee orchid employs a sexual deception scenario to lure male bumble bees to its flower. Do you think the bumble bee orchid perceives the difference between male and female bees?

Total respondents = 73

2 respondents skipped

64 respondents answered Yes = 87.84 %

9 respondents answered No = 12.33 %

Question (6)

The bumble bee orchid employs a sexual deception scenario to lure male bumble bees to its flower. Do you think this shows ability to plan and reason?

Total respondents = 74

1 respondent skipped

45 respondents answered Yes = 60.81 %

29 respondents answered No = 39.19 %

Question (7)

The bumble bee orchid knows how to replicate the sex pheromone of the female bumble bee. Do you think this shows knowledge of chemistry and intelligence?

Total respondents = 73

2 respondents skipped

47 respondents answered Yes = 64.38 %

26 respondents answered No = 35.62 %

Question (8)

Do you think the bumble bee orchid is aware of its environment?

Total respondents = 74

1 respondent skipped

69 respondents answered Yes = 93.24 %

5 respondents answered No = 6.76 %

(Plant Awareness)

Q 1 If a plant emits an alarm pheromone that calls an insect to its aid, do you think the plant knows this specific insect exists?

75 Respondents
60 Yes 15 No
80/20

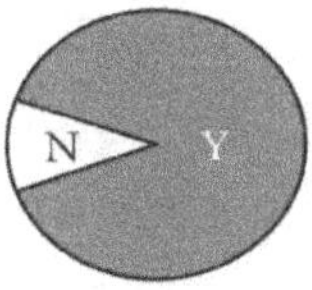

Q 2 Is it logical to extrapolate that if a plant knows one insect in its environment that it knows others?

74 Respondents / 1 Skipped
65 Yes 9 No
87.84/12.16

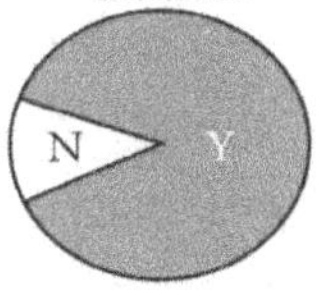

Q 3 A tomato worm is eating a tomato plant. The plant emits an alarm pheromone to attract the horned worm wasp which kills the tomato worm and lays its eggs in it. Do you think the tomato plant knows this when it is calling the horned worm wasp for help?

75 Respondents
57 Yes 18 No
76/18

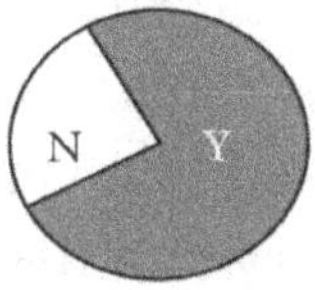

Q 4 Do you think the tomato plant knows it is attracting the horned wasp?

75 Respondents
55 Yes 20 No
73.33/26.67

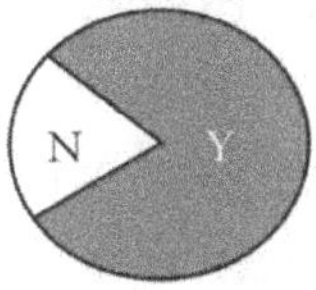

Q 5 It has been proven that the bumble bee orchid employs a sexual deception scenario to lure male bumble bees to its flower. Do you think the bumble bee orchid perceives the difference between male and female bees?

73 Respondents / 3 Skipped
64 Yes 9 No
87.84/12.33

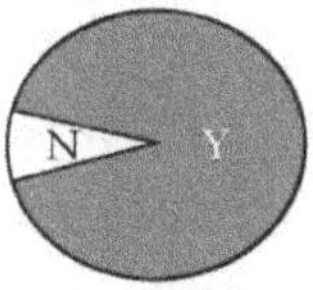

Q 6 The bumble bee orchid employs a sexual deception scenario to lure male bumble bees to its flower. Do you think this shows ability to plan and reason?

74 Respondents / 1 Skipped
45 Yes 29 No
60.81/39.19

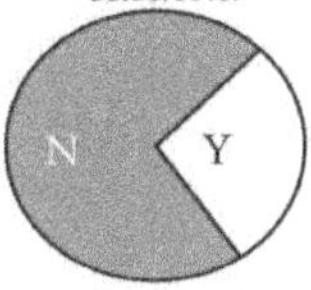

Q 7 The bumble bee orchid knows how to replicate the sex pheromone of the female bumble bee. Do you think this shows knowledge of chemistry and intelligence?

73 Respondents / 2 Skipped
47 Yes 26 No
64.38/35.62

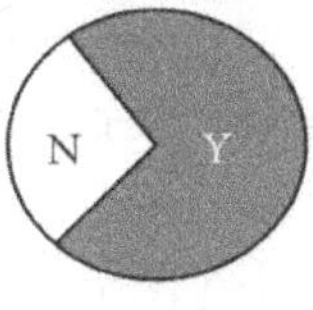

Q 8 Do you think the bumble bee orchid is aware of its environment?

74 Respondents / 1 Skipped
69 Yes 5 No
93.24/6.76

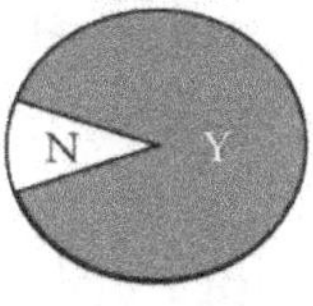

Why does a plant evolve with respect to color, shape, and size? Logically, it must create advantages for the plant to do so--otherwise, why do it? It is illogical for a plant to alter its shape, size or color if doing so does not provide an advantage. It is apparent there are intelligent and organizing Photon Information Expressions which are present in all living things. I believe Photon Information Expressions direct and promote the survival and propagation of a species via DNA and environmental factors. These environmental factors can mitigate or completely reverse these basic DNA instructions. It is my assertion that your Reality Replication Template, in conjunction with DNA, epigenetic data, and quantum intent create you. It is also observed that sentience and sapience is demonstrated as sensory awareness (See Examples of Plant Intelligence). Lastly, it is observed that some plants exhibit and implement survival strategies that are intelligent responses directed at their environments (See Examples of Plant Intelligence).

Does a plant know what is in its environment? Can various plants make conscious choices based on this information? Empirical scientific observation indicates, yes (See Examples of Plant Intelligence). This assertion is supported by the observation that conscious adaptations are made by plants based on sensory information collected from their environment (See Examples of Plant Intelligence). Why would a plant emit a pheromone that attracts a specific insect to it, if it did not know that insect existed? How could it? Why would a plant evolve with external genitalia that were a specific color, size, and shape if it did not aide in the fertilization process by attracting pollinators to itself? A belief that this process just evolved that way provides no credible evidence to support their assertion.

It is logical to assert the bumble bee orchids and other plants "know" the specific insects which exist in their environment. Out of the thousands of insects that live in their environment, a specific insect, in this case the male bumble bee, is selected as the preferred aide in a plant's quest for survival and biological reproduction. Additionally, the ruse or con game implemented by the bumble bee orchid has proven successful (an ability to think and reason!). This is evidenced by its longevity. If this were not the case, the bumble bee orchid would be forced to adapt a different strategy to survive or experience a death-transition, or even a life extinction event.

Which is a more logical and reasonable statement: (1) The bumble bee orchid collects sensory data obtained from its environment utilizing an intelligent systematic process for the purpose of incorporating this data toward survival and evolvement. (2) The bumble bee orchid evolves not being aware of any of its sensory data. It actively collects data and interacts with its environment. However, during the experiencing of these data, it is not aware of its survival equation. Statement (2) is a blind exclusion of logical cognitive data, a System of Interference. It is ill-logical to assert the bumble bee orchid exhibits awareness during the collection of sensory data and then assert there is no awareness associated with this process.

Many plants create symbiotic relationships (See Examples of Plant Intelligence) which will entice or lure an insect to visit a specific plant. Some plants use sweet nectar. Some, like the bumble bee orchid, use deception. Still others use symbiotic relationships with animals (See Examples of Plant Intelligence). Phyto-biology and molecular biology are continually recording and expanding their research regarding this observation of communication with plants (See Examples of Plant Intelligence). However, researchers are reluctant to include many observations due to the possibility of being ostracized in the scientific community. This is an example of Systems of Interference and an example of the old "square peg in a round hole example A quantitative methodology is not all encompassing, and it omits qualitative data (Cognition, non-local observations, etc.) observed to be present. Without the use of a "systems integration" approach many of the obvious observations cannot be included, thus exhibiting Systems of Interference, and creating bias.

Medicinal plants support the self-healing experience. This is an experience that has been documented for thousands of years! Reconnect with this intelligence and utilize plants to support your ability to self-heal.

An extraordinary example of plant intelligence (sentience, sapience, and quantum signature) is the Bumble Bee Orchid (Ophrys-Bombyliflora). We will elaborate on this in the next chapter. This type of awareness and perception observed in plants is more than most humans are aware of.

Chapter 10

"The bumble bee orchid is creating its own reality."
—Dr. G. Munger

The Bumble Bee Orchid (Ophrys-Bombyliflora)

This chapter will help explain why "live" intelligent plants that utilize Photon Information Expressions support the self-healing of humans—they, too, have varying degrees of intelligence and awareness!

The foundations on which many of the conclusions this chapter comes to are based on the published works of Trewavas [1] and Cvrckova, Lipovska, & Zarsky [2], 2009. (These folks are brilliant and worth the read.) The bumble bee orchid, my chosen example, utilizes intelligence (quantum phyto-sapience) in its unique approach toward propagation of itself. The bumble bee orchid demonstrates the ability to (1) observe quantum waves of possibilities and collapse those waves into particles of reality using intent; just like humans (2) utilize a sense of sight or photonic image detection, yes it can see colors and its environment (3) it employs reason (4) recognizes the difference between male and female bumble bees (5) keenly understands the sexual reproduction instincts of bumble bees (6) specifically selected the male bumble bee to aid as a pollination vector (7) exhibits intelligent decision making which can be observed when it morphs part of its labellum to resemble a 3-dimensional shape of a female bumble bee (8) recognizes the shape of the bumble bee and remembers (utilizes memory) of how to reproduce it.

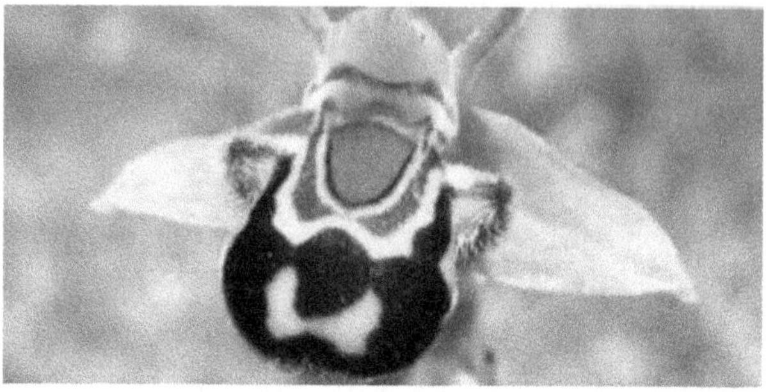

(Bumble Bee Orchid (Ophrys-Bombyliflora), Pinterest.com)

(9) creates a sophisticated version of a female virgin sex pheromone [2] which is emitted into the air to attract the male bumble bee to the orchid.

These observations indicate the bumble bee orchid utilizes the same sensory data exhibited by humans to collect and analyze data. The logical explanation of these actions is the bumble bee orchid employs reasoning **(rSd + MA + Res = SA)** which is consistent with the luring and attracting of the male bumble bee to its flower. What I mean by this is, the bumble bee orchid scams or tricks the male Bumble Bee into visiting its location. During this process the male bumble bee detects a version of the female bumble bee sex pheromone which has been emitted into the air and flies to the source of the emission, a version that is close enough to the real sex pheromone to fool the male bumble bee (in fact researchers are finding the male bumble bees prefer the copy). The male bumble bee is presented with a 3-Dimensional physical representation of the female bumble bee. This is a replica of the female bumble bee, in color. It is logical to extrapolate that the bumble bee orchid must have a way of sensing photonic images in the electromagnetic spectrum (sight). The bumble bee orchid can depict what the female bumble bee looks like to the male bumble bee and is able to engineer a 3-dimensional representation. Without this ability to observe or detect photonic images of the female bumble bee, the bumble bee orchid would not be able to create a likeness. The fact that a physical 3-D representation of the female bumble bee exists is an example of intelligent intent and design consistent with **(D) + (ROR) = Proof.** This is complex cognitive behavior (engineering). This is sapient behavior.

Another example of intelligence exhibited by the bumble bee orchid is the manufacture or replication of a female bumble bee's sex pheromone (variation). This is comprised of a complex chemical composition of pyrazine. [3] The bumble bee orchid's inclusion of this pheromone exhibits reason and shows knowledge of its environment and the sexual habits of bumble bees. It would be illogical and a waste of resources for the bumble bee orchid to create a sex pheromone to attract the male bumble bee if it did not know this aspect of the bumble bee's mating habits would lure a male bumble bee to its location. The inclusion of this sex pheromone with the 3-Dimemsional color representation of the female bumble bee is an elaborate deception. [2]

This type of reasoning indicates analysis, memory, and exhibits engineering and artistic interpretation. The analysis utilized by the bumble bee orchid exhibits the ability to discern the difference between male and female bumble bees and displays an understanding of their sexual instincts. Furthermore, the bumble bee orchid's sapient ability exhibits a strategy or plan to use these creations to augment their pollination process. This adaptation by the bumble bee orchid exhibits complex planning skills and an obvious understanding of how to lure the male bumble bee using the scent of a female bumble bee. The bumble bee orchid exhibits the use of memory, reason, photonic reception of holographic images and "intent" to accomplish this remarkable strategy.

The bumble bee orchid is keenly aware of its environment. It analyzes and perceives information about the bumble bee, [2]and this awareness exhibits an understanding not previously thought to exist in the bumble bee orchid and is one of the reasons for this analysis. This type of sensory data could not have been included in a quantitative research model. The bumble bee orchid can synthesize a version of the sex pheromone of a female virgin bumble bee. [1], [2] This logically requires a sample of the pheromone and more importantly, a sophisticated knowledge of how to replicate it. This chemical awareness is combined with a phenomenal ability to accurately recall this data. This is evidenced by the "existence" of the simulated sex pheromone. The bumble bee orchid exhibits a memory process which can recall data in a remarkable manner. The bumble bee memory process is consistent with its degree of sapience and consistent with its specific needs. It is logical to conclude a female bumble bee sex pheromone sample is extracted from contact with the female bumble bee (it would need to obtain a sample to replicate it). This exhibits awareness of its environment and the ability to discern specific chemical compounds. How this is accomplished will be the focus of another paper. The fact that the chemical compound exists in a material form is proof it was synthesized. The formula synthesized by the bumble bee orchid must be "exacting enough" to fool the male bumble bee into thinking he is interacting with a female for the purpose of copulation and or reproduction. This logically requires an exacting breakdown of the female bumble bee sex pheromone. This pharmaceutical process [4] is most complex. Even more remarkable is that the bumble bee orchid must utilize constituents that are only available in its environment to accomplish this and use its own physical structure as a laboratory. This process exhibits the bumble bee orchid's ability to chemically analyze and manufacture a replica of the female bumble bee's sex pheromone. This is an ability which shows sophisticated understanding of biochemistry. [5]

It is not the focus of this paper to investigate how the bumble bee orchid replicates the required constituents to manufacture the female bumble bee sex pheromone. All that is required is that the pheromone needs to be present and quantifiable. If constituents of the female bumble bee sex pheromone are not innate substances available to the bumble bee orchid, then logically, the constituents must come from somewhere in the environment. Bio-transmutation is one possibility (although not well documented). These abilities of the bumble bee orchid indicate an exceptional awareness of itself, reasoning and intelligent design.

Included in this observation is the logic that if a bumble bee orchid can *see* or detect holographic images of one insect, then logically it can see other insects. This detection ability would logically apply to other aspects of its environment as well. This observation by the bumble bee orchid exhibits awareness and intelligent design. As astonishing as this is in and of itself, the fact that the bumble bee orchid accomplishes this is evidence of its ability to detect and select quantum waves of possibility into intended particles of reality. ***The bumble bee orchid is creating its own reality*** (quantum phyto-sapeince). This capability was previously and exclusively deemed to be a human attribute [6] (anthropomorphic). It is important to remember what is required for this to occur. When one employs the logical use of cognitive observations with material observations (quantitative and qualitative methodologies) of the bumble bee orchid, an inescapable conclusion presents itself. This flower exhibits intelligent design, consistency, sapience, and quantum expression of awareness—organized intelligence.

Plant intelligence exists! Do you think it would be advantageous to enlist the help of a live plant that is already being used by the medical community to support your self-healing? I do! Take astragalus for example: Astragalus exhibits anti-microbial, anti-bacterial and anti-fungal properties, among others. Herbalists and compounding pharmacies already use this herb to treat a variety of presentations. I believe the scientific community should be trying to understand this plant by employing an in-vivo approach (live specimen). The focus of this analysis being "augmentation" of the already existing properties of astragalus. I believe we can introduce DNA, via blood, saliva, etc. to a research specimen of live astragalus with the goal being a "molecular hello", so to speak. One of our goals would be to create a symbiotic relationship with this plant. These possibilities are pregnant and waiting. It is my observation that all a plant wants from humans is to feed it, tend it, love it, and allow it to continue its LIFE path. However, now that we know some plants are sapient, maybe this relationship can reveal much more.

Would this live approach have a positive impact toward supporting self-healing? I believe yes. Imagine experimenting with live plants that could provide their subjective feed-back. Our goal should be to use "quantum intent" to augment our awareness of the healing abilities already exhibited in astragalus.

Plants support self-healing awareness in an intelligent, organized manner! Most people are not aware of this aspect of their interactions with them. In fact, we have been utilizing dead specimens and still experiencing healing results. In the next chapter we will elaborate on some of the observations associated with plants—it is no wonder they produce such a positive effect on humans.

Chapter 11

"Everyone has to seek nature for himself."
—Masanobu Fukuoka

"An intelligent and organized live field expression is not exclusively exhibited by humans—it is the same live field expression observed in all forms of life."
—Dr. G. Munger

Sentience and Sapience of Plants

As previously discussed in Chapter 8, unclear or ambiguous definitions create a thought process that utilizes Systems of Interference. Even more problematic is that your thought process considers the definition factual! *Any believed definition always creates an impact on your Reality Replication Template.* To that end, utilizing only human data sources limits your choice of information possibilities. Healthy plants are a reliable resource to support self-healing. The use of "live" plants has been observed in human and other life forms for thousands of years. Become aware of plants and their properties. Live intelligent plants are underused by humans. Using "intention", live plants can be used to create or augment the quantified properties identified in them that currently mitigate or eliminate disease. For instance, the plant astragalus, mentioned before has properties identified as anti-bacterial, anti-fungal and anti-inflammatory; it is also observed to boost the immune system. These properties were identified using an in-vitro (dead specimen) approach. Imagine using an in-vivo (live specimen) approach and asking (intending) the astragalus plant to augment its already identified properties! Is this far-fetched? It works on humans.

Let us examine some definitions and expand some of them to include plants.

Sentient is defined by Merriam-Webster dictionary [1] as "responsive to or conscious of sense impressions." Does my equation, sensory data + modified awareness (RRT) = Sentience **(Sd + MA = S)** fulfill this definition for plants? It works for humans.

Sapient is defined by Merriam-Webster dictionary as "possessing or expressing great sagacity." [2] Does this equation, sensory data + modified awareness (RRT) + reason + memory = Sapience **(Sd + MA + Res + rSd = SA)** fulfill this definition? Again, it works for humans.

The understanding of sentience and sapience must logically include other animals and plants. If plants or other non-human animals exhibit the **same** criteria required to be considered sentient or sapient in humans, then they are sentient or sapient—simple logic. If an organism exhibits the same traits considered sentient or sapient for humans, then we can say this organism possess one or both qualities. If we do not apply the same definition criteria to all examples, then we have employed Systems of Interference and anthropomorphic bias. *An intelligent and organized live field expression is not exclusively exhibited by humans—it is the same live field expression observed in all forms of LIFE.* This is a good observation. With this understanding I believe we can augment the effectiveness of medicinal plants using live field expressions and quantum thought expressions.

We can expand on this further to include other life forms which can collapse quantum waves of possibility into particles of reality using their *intent*—remember, many plants exhibit sentience and/or sapience, like the bumble bee orchid.

I have coined a few definitions that will help clarify the awareness properties in plants.

Phyto-Sentience and Phyto-Sapience

Phyto-sentience, coined by me, is defined as a plant's ability to be aware of and consciously interact with its environment. This definition is based on the definition of the word "sentience". According to Merriam Wester [3] "...responsive to or conscious of sense impressions, sentient beings, aware, finely sensitive in perception or feeling." This new definition is required since there is no definition for plant sentience (phyto-sentience). Sensory data combined with a plant's modified awareness equals sentience **(Sd + MA = S).**

Phyto-sapience, coined by me, includes phyto-sentience's definition and is defined as a plant's ability to be aware of and consciously interact with its environment, and it exhibits the ability to think, reason and has the ability to store and recall data at a later (memory) time. There has been much controversy attached to this subject (plant intelligence) due to the unclear methodology utilized and ambiguous definitions applied to reach these current conclusions. Phyto-sapience utilizes the same criteria required to determine sapience in humans. Sensory data combined with modified awareness that utilizes reason and memory data which can include repeated sensory data results, is sapience **(Sd + MA + Res + rSd = SA).**

There have been numerous studies compiled on plant intelligence. [4] However, most of these observations were documented using limited scientific inquiry or a stand-alone methodology. As mentioned before, this is utilizing definitions not adequate to analyze *all* the observed data. The predominate view formed within a framework of a reductionistic quantitative science methodology exhibits Systems of Interference when it excludes pertinent data (non-local data) which is present during an analysis. By employing a cognitive model (qualitative methodology), logical conclusions can be included utilizing specific examples of material data. Material data combined with non-material data requires the merging of two or more scientific research models. This is the systems integration approach needed to account for data that cannot be included in conclusions derived by a stand-alone quantitative model.

It goes without saying that all data must be accounted for. Any data that is observed but omitted during research skews the results and confers bias (Systems of Interference). A cognitive science observation combined with linear scientific observations produces a systems integration approach and provides a superior model for understanding the non-linear as well as the linear aspects of plants (See Chapter 10, Bumble Bee Orchid). Plants use many of the same senses that humans utilize to collect data. Plants make decisions and choose the best option to employ for their species-specific circumstances. The important observation here is not to confuse phyto-sentience with phyto-sapience.

Quantum Phyto-Sapience

Quantum Phyto-Sapience, coined by me, is the ability of a phyto-sapient plant to utilize "intention" combined with observations, to collapse quantum waves of possibility into particles of reality. Pertinent to this discussion on plants is a definition describing what is required in quantum physics to collapse quantum waves of possibility into particles of reality. According to Astrophysicist Dr. Amit Goswami, [5] "In quantum physics, objects are depicted as possibilities (a possibility wave); yet when an observer observes these possibilities they collapse into an actuality." Some sapient plants can see, are aware of their environment, and utilize intention to interact with their environment. It is important to be aware of your own intent when compiling data since this, too, can influence data collection. According to the late scientist, Stephen Hawking, "A researcher's intent can skew the results of an experiment." [6] This chapter's intent is to provide evidence of plant intelligence. It re-enforces the idea that plants (bumble bee orchids) exhibit the capacity to collapse quantum waves of possibility into particles of reality. It is our responsibility to make sure when we are observing this process taking place in plants, that we stay constantly aware of the Systems of Interference which confer anthropomorphic bias.

My example of quantum phyto-sapience, which occurs in the bumble bee orchid, exhibits the utilization of the same sensory data required by humans to achieve a collapse of a quantum wave of possibility into a particle of reality. This means the bumble bee orchid must be able to be aware of and consciously interact with its environment, have a quantum sense of self, and create its own reality. This investigation of the bumble bee orchid supports this logic. The Bumble Bee orchid also exhibits the ability to reason and demonstrates the capacity for memory of data which can be recalled later. Sapient abilities have been exhibited and demonstrated by the bumble bee orchid.

All plants are sentient, and many are sapient. Some plants have the same quantum abilities that humans do. Wouldn't it be logical to entertain the thought of enlisting quantum phyto-sapient plants to help support our self-healing awareness? Live plants have the potential to address aspects of healing that dead-transitioned plants cannot (Photon Information Expressions no longer exist in dead-transitioned plant, so we cannot communicate with them). Plants support humans and all life on earth—hopefully, a perpetual observation. In our next chapter we will show you how to support your own self-healing.

Chapter 12

"Humankind has not woven the web of LIFE. We are but one thread within it. Whatever we do to the web, we do to ourselves. All things are bound together. All things are connected."—Chief Seattle

How to Support Self-Healing

We humans can use all the help we can get! Constant imbalances like intrusions of environmental toxins, nutritional deficiencies, psychological imbalances and an invincible ignorance dictated by economic, political and medical bias are but a few of the reasons "un-consciousness" the human species. These imbalances contribute to and affect your personal experience of health. This observation affects the overall health of all humans or the Group Reality Replication Template of our species' health.

I cannot believe how many books, good ones, are written on the nutritional aspects of health. Yet, few humans heed their advice! What kind of GRRT is that?

Nutrition is an essential aspect of self-healing. Each person metabolizes food in their own way—it is not the same for everyone. What are your individual specific needs to metabolize food? If you do not know what your norm is, you are unaware of the specific mind and body requirements that can maximize your self-healing potential. The blind spot is a type of un-awareness that lets you assume your generalized diet is adequate. You do not want adequate, you want optimal. I believe "adequate" has a negative impact on the effectiveness of nutrition. For example, a balanced diet comprised of vegetables, fruit, protein, adequate hydration, exercise, etc. is promoted in most of the nutritional books I have read. This is a good start, but…

Guess what? There is no such thing as a general nutritional diet that fits everyone. You need to identify your *own* specific nutritional dietary needs. I suggest enlisting the help of a licensed nutritionist who will work with you and your doctor of choice. Some people are allergic to certain foods yet are not aware of this! For instance, an allergy does not necessarily have to be severe or life threatening. Sometimes people don't even know they are having an allergic reaction to specific food because the reaction is small and they have not developed enough "healing awareness" (they do not know what their normal health status feels like) to detect it or remove it (Or, they detect it, but brush it aside as insignificant—lack of awareness). Take the time to find out for yourself what *you* can eat and what you cannot. Most professional nutritionists will help you with this or they can refer you to someone who can.

Are you using a generalized exercise program?

Guess what? There is no such thing as a general exercise program that fits everyone. This is so obvious that it should not have to be listed here. Orthopedic presentations, illness, weakness, psychological perceptions, and one's general overall fitness needs to be considered. This will affect one's choice of an exercise program. When it comes to exercise programs, consult as many professionals as you deem necessary to come up with a personalized exercise program that is right for you. Remember to include someone who can counsel you regarding *your* psychological perceptions of exercise as well. Keep in mind the objective is a balanced routine you can replicate, not preparing for an Olympic gold medal. I saw an older couple (in their 90s) that had a daily work out that is worth mentioning. They laid down on their backs on the floor and rocked their legs and arms back and forth. They never left the floor, and they received a great and safe workout. **Exercise every day, like the rest of the animals on earth do**. Get to know your body.

Lymph does not have an organ like the heart to pump lymph through your body. *Movement is required.* Make your exercise routine a social gathering (if possible) containing smiles, laughter, and conversations (think of sharing, not belittling others—yes it affects your workout).

Guess what? There is no such thing as a general psychological profile that fits everyone. Fear, psycho-social experiences and much more affect your ability to engage in healthy eating or living. I have seen many patients over the years. During this time, I was able to recognize many Reality Replication Templates (even before I knew of their existence). Ralph Waldo Emerson is quoted as noting the same thing, "Who you are speaks so loudly I can't hear what you're saying." One such reoccurring scenario was a patient who presented as clinically obese.

I believe obesity is a difficult subject to bridge with most patients. It requires increased sensitivity and awareness to speak with a patient about this. If you lovingly tell them they are dangerously overweight, a common reply they have rehearsed well will be expounded upon. Most of the time they do not come back since once again, they are being asked to fail. Most of these patients cannot help themselves, so they hide from me and develop an RRT which allows them hide from themselves. This cannot be achieved by anyone, if all I get is 7 minutes with a patient; the industry standard. We need to create an atmosphere that is without judgement and psychologically safe. This can occur once the patient becomes self-aware. The primary concentration is on helping them attain "awareness". I have learned that without doing this first, you are asking them to do the impossible. If they could lose weight, they would have done it long ago. More importantly, without awareness, they *cannot see* their health is being interfered with by their Reality Replication Template. All they know is they are overweight and have tried multiple times to lose this weight. They do not know how to change their eating habits. They experience failure after failure until they give up. Then their wall of fear goes up. Their RRT is, "This can't be changed" and leave me alone. How can someone know they are dangerously overweight, yet not want to heal this condition? Unawareness of your RRT will do it every time. It has been my experience that most of these patients have a "story" to validate their individual specific version of their Reality Replication Template regarding their state of health (not just obesity)! Guess what? These folks are *unaware* of their Reality Replication Template which resists or prohibits CHANGE. Additionally, you cannot change something if you do not know it exists—an impenetrable ignorance.

Do not exclude yourself from this observation. As discussed in this book, most people are not even aware of their Reality Replication Template. For instance, these folks know their (insert any detrimental habit here) is bad for them, yet they keep repeating the unconscious behavior. Being unaware of your RRT, makes you reactive instead of interactive. If you are not aware of self-conditioning, how can you ask for help? As previously mentioned, this is due to unawareness of their RRT—**they only let information into their reality which supports their RRT, even if it is detrimental behavior**. They do not realize that a "perception" of their self even exists. These people *literally* cannot hear this advice. Their tympanic membrane is vibrating, but the sound wave interpretation will only support your reality. It has been my experience that very few patients want to talk about how to change. They are extremely uncomfortable talking about repeating what they have already experienced as a failure. Their response is (in general), "You don't understand." This is a heart-breaking exclamation of emotion for me. They are, in effect, telling me they are not aware of any options. They tell me, "I have tried many, many times to change, stop, or heal, I just can't." Their RRT is "I just can't." I continually endeavor to establish love and trust. Unfortunately, sometimes their shield is too strong. Unfortunately, only they can make this change.

Individual specific awareness is where their emphasis should be. *The wonderful part of this is that it is non-invasive and creates the change desired.* It is yours for the asking. Wouldn't self-healing awareness help this presentation? Would not knowing how YOU create your own Reality Replication Template establish a new perspective? If you can help one person with this understanding they can, *for first time in their life,* change to a balanced health presentation. They can create effective strategies directed at self-healing awareness and finally find the person they have always been. This is how anyone and everyone does it.

All healing is self-healing. Self-healing awareness creates or promotes individual specific healing (It is *you* who helps or hinder this process). This "self-realized" healing of you creates the awareness to heal and balance all aspects of life—not just your health. When I realized this for the first time, I just laughed at myself. How could this be so simple and yet I was not aware of this? It does not matter how many times you have failed; you are learning you now have new knowledge and perception of how this whole thing works. This "quantum state of knowing" empowers healing within the physical and mental bodies. Healing fields of information are requested from LIFE. Photon Information Expressions carry this data flow through all the variations of "life"—it is *you* who mitigates this process. Please remember, this is not an all or nothing experience. Your healing awareness is achieved in varying degrees (Remember, you already do it). Choose to become aware of YOU—your Reality Replication Template. All that is required is "intention" to do so, and a sense of humor (Ha!).

An important aspect of self-healing, your gift to humanity and the environment, is that it can help heal others. Additionally, anyone I have ever met that gained this "awareness" always helps others struggling to find themselves. Wouldn't you help someone stuck in the same type of unawareness that you experienced? As mentioned before, all humans affect their environment. This is expressed as a "collective knowledge" and created by projecting their individual specific interpretation of their data into the previously mentioned Total Information Continuum. Arlene Lorrance is the first person quoted to have said, "Be the change you want to see happen." [1] Self-healing is the conscious path back to a balanced you and a balanced world.

Quantum healing awareness will help you heal your-self. This awareness automatically helps provide pro-conscious feed-back towards healing everything. Each healthy, aware human contributes to the overall healthy balance of everything. *Yes, you are critical to this process.* It can be compared to a large clean-up project. Start anywhere with the intent to clean-up. With this awareness and persistence, it will eventually become clean. When "you" pick-up a piece of paper for example, especially one that you didn't throw on the ground, you have exhibited "awareness" of your environment. When you clean debris from a small stream which someone else left, you have also exhibited "awareness", and when you love yourself, this too is awareness.

Now, apply this to *yourself* and experience your awareness. It does not matter where you start, just start.

Awareness is available to anyone, anywhere, any race, any time. Reach out with intention to change—you will not be disappointed.

Unawareness is also a Reality Replication Template. It is an unawareness of your Reality Replication Templates, Lock-on Lock-out principles, and Systems of Interference. We have all experienced and are susceptible to this type of un-consciousness, me included. However, with self-awareness we can CHANGE who we are anytime we wish. In fact, self-awareness is a quantum leap toward consciousness. *Awareness is always available to those who ask for it.* How can you comprehend what is being said here if you are in a state of invincible ignorance or have an impenetrable RRT shield? Intention to do so is the only way. This book has shown you ways of detecting who you are. You are (RIGHT NOW!) learning a new perspective of "how you become you". It does not matter how you got to your current imbalance. All that is required is you must *intend* any change you want to experience—remember, you already do it. It just has not been pointed out to you before. The "change experience" is observed by who you are right now! This person was created by you. All I am doing is pointing this out. Reality Replication Templates can and do change all the time. Lock-on lock-out principle is real. Systems of Interference permeate our existence. RRTs and GRRTs are continuously being created. Let me help you become you. All that is required is choosing to become aware of how you do what you do.

Start small. By experimenting with your awareness, you will change the way you experience your reality. This will give you evidence of change and it will propel you forward to consciousness. However, you also have the option to continue down your current path—even if this path is not working for you. This is not a bad thing; it is an unaware thing. It is doing the best you can with what you know. However, I have introduced you to a new approach which works for ANYONE that intends to change. I can only show you, not do it for you. I am willing to help in any way I can. Look for the person inside yourself who has always been there, the person you want to be again. I promise that person is still there.

There are many medical modalities that can help with self-healing. I have listed some of them in the next chapter. Additionally, immediately following the next chapter is the experiment I conducted which supports the existence of a "general information" understanding of data exhibited by the human species, our GRRT.

Chapter 13

"Intuition will tell the thinking mind where to look next."—Jonas Salk

Types of Medicine Practices

The following list of medical modalities are but a sampling of the medical treatment interpretations which exist in the world today. Each appears to understand part of the healing equation yet falls short as a *complete* strategy for creating health and curing disease. This is evidenced by the fact that humans all over the world are incorporating multiple medical treatments and maintenance therapies with multiple doctors, because they are not achieving the healing results they want. [1] Why would they do this if one specific medicine were the total treatment package? Obviously, they would not. Medicine is still trial and error. We must pierce the shield of ego, economics and the ignorance which exists in a "my way only" scenario. Together, we can integrate all medicine to create a (Group Reality Replication Template). This inability to consolidate or integrate medicine is due to Systems of Interference—mostly ego and economic intrusion. Until the day when the entire global medical community integrates all viable "types of medicine practices" into ONE understanding, not just an individual interpretation, we will remain fragmented and searching. Undoubtedly, when this integration occurs it will reflect a pre-disposition to rely on "self-awareness" and "self-healing" as a means of affecting change.

We will continue our research toward a unified understanding of medicine even it requires using "fragments of truth" gleaned from the various medicines, researchers and healing modalities practiced all over the world.

This "fragmented truth "observation implores you to employ reason and consult with your doctor, universities, researchers, healers, other licensed health professionals and those which have "survived" the same diagnosis you are currently experiencing. I believe this should be done prior to choosing a medical treatment strategy. However, you make up your own mind. You can never have too much scientific information, emotional support, or love!

Please remember, no one should know you better than you. Be your own primary collector of information concerning your physical body, your mental expression and your God or quantum belief experience—this is something only you can do.

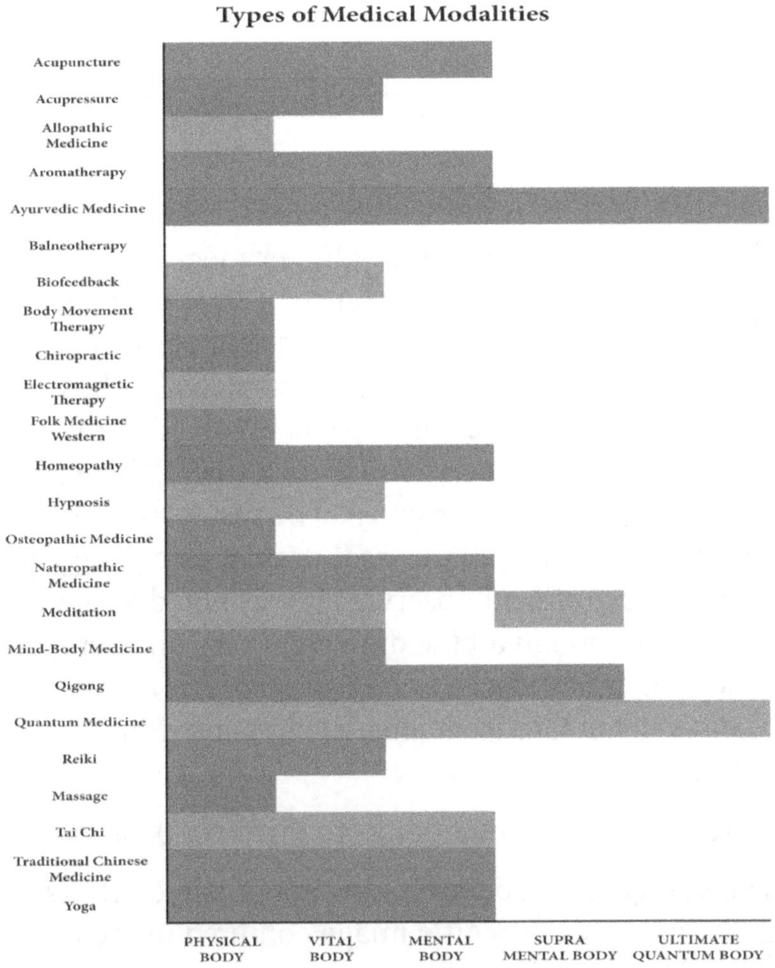

The above (5) categories, are observations of (1) material physical body and of (4) non-material expressions of awareness fields.

Chapter 14

"Trust shows the way."—Hildegard of Bingen

Subjective Memory Experiment

This "Subjective Memory Experiment" provides data to support the existence of an intelligent quantum field of data that is continually updated and accessed by humans and could conceivably be used by other life forms. The participants involved in this experiment were instructed to "draw a tree". This was all the information they were given. The results of this experiment indicated all the trees drawn were different. However, a significant observation was noted in these results. Even though all the drawings were different, they were still interpreted as a tree. *A generalized agreement was observed;* a Group Reality Replication Template (GRRT).

1. A tree means different things to different people.

2. The ability to reproduce a likeness of a tree differs with the individual specific image conjured in their minds and their artistic ability to reproduce this image on a piece of paper.

3. Note how many different types of trees were submitted.

4. A general image and definition of a tree can be extrapolated for each example submitted. This is true even though most of these examples are not real examples of trees. This is an example of photonic

encoding of data which is modified by your Reality Replication Template and your individual specific ability to replicate a perceived image. This creates a *generally agreed upon* group human species perception of this image.

Tree Image Experiment

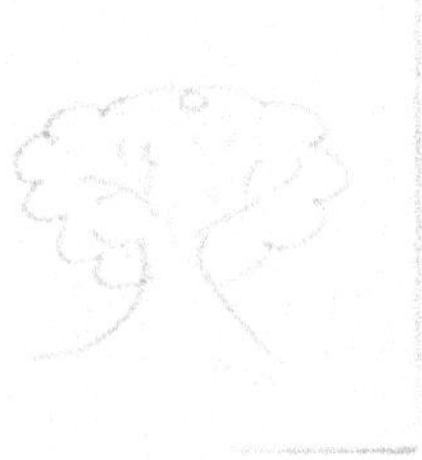
Image #1

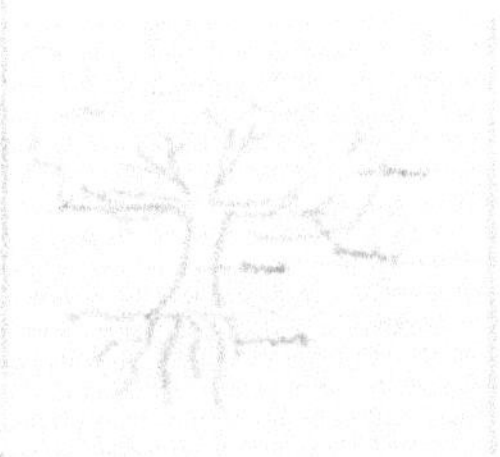
Image #2

Image #3

Image #4

Image #5

Image #6

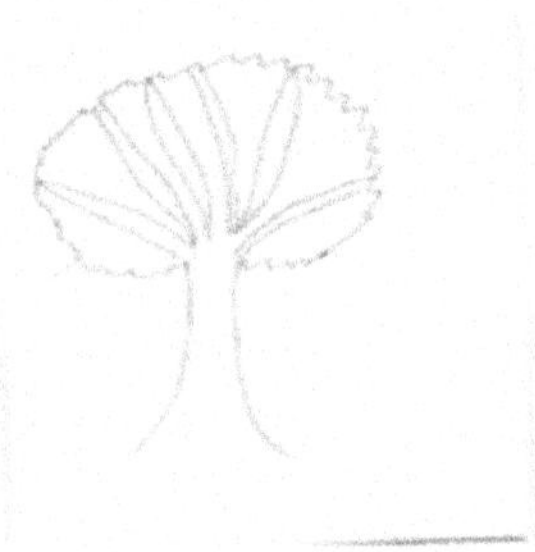
Image # 7

Image #8

Image #9

Image # 10

Image #11

Image #12

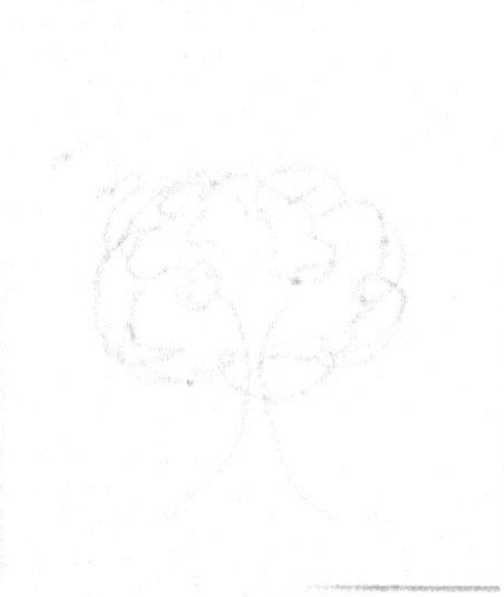

Image #13

Image #14

Image #15

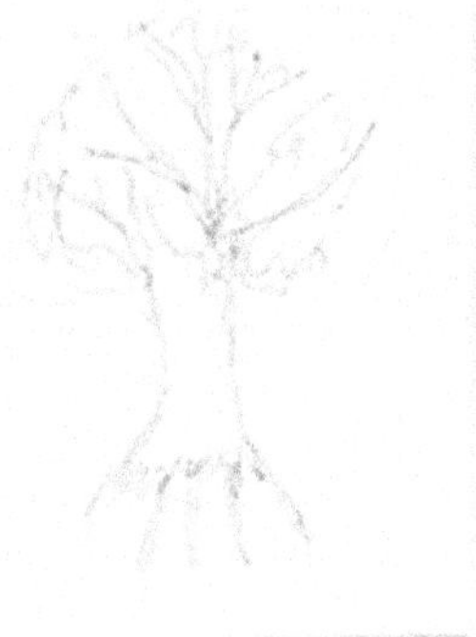

Image #16

Image #17

Image #18

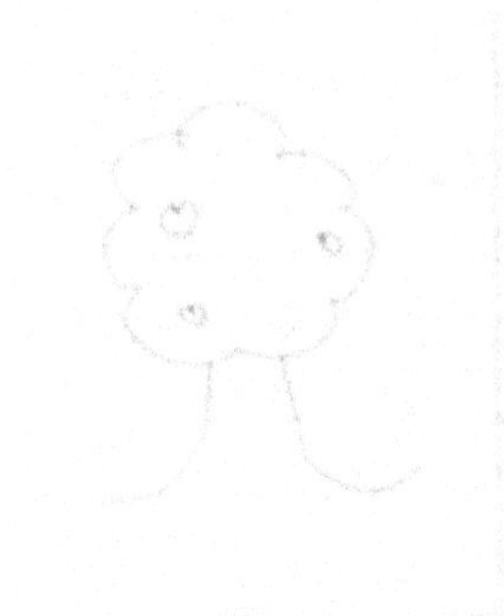

Image # 19

Image #20

Image #21

Image #22

Image #23

Image #24

Image #25

(There were actually 116 images, but I decided 25 examples were enough to include here—the rest of the images are similar to these 25). Try this yourself, there won't be a duplicate. The results of this experiment conclude photonic representations of objects can be observed as a "universal image language" that creates a generalized *meaning* understood in all cultures (it transcends languages). The trees drawn by these participants are individual representations of trees images. I believe the human species' shares a general information collective which is part of LIFE's Total Information Continuum data base. This database establishes and provides a general understanding of what a tree is.

If the people of any culture (even if they have different languages) viewed these "tree images" they could identifiy the drawings as trees. They are photonic representations of trees as "thought expressions" experienced in the mind and are generally accepted as images of a tree—a universal language.

Chapter 15

"Only you can find you."—Dr. G. Munger

Analyze, Adapt, and Evolve

As previously discussed, I believe all humans experience life as an interpretation of their self-created Reality Replication Template. I believe humans continuously upload and share information contained in a Total Information Continuum database. This database is a combination of all data which has been collected by humans and other life forms (live expressions). I believe this "upload of data" is achieved by utilizing Photon Information Expressions (an extension of the original LIFE) which continually provide individual specific data to the Total Information Continuum. When this information field is accessed by you for the purpose of "identifying" an image of something, it provides a *more* "expanded interpretation" or generally accepted interpretation of that image—as evidenced in my tree drawing experiment. An image conveys more data than just uttering the word tree.

So, how does one become informed, knowledgeable, and aware? You are already learning the answer to this question. You just *intend* to learn! Knowledge can only be accumulated by you using your individual subjective experience or Reality Replication Template. Knowledge coupled with perception is awareness **(K + P = A)**. It is the awareness of this template coupled with the intent to use it, which provides a desired change.

As part of this process, we will be required to develop a way of discerning logical and accurate information utilizing an awareness of Systems of Interference we can detect. Science and history books change continually. However, not before they impart data to you—in many cases, incorrect data. This is the reason material data and logical extrapolation of non-material data are of such importance. How can you be aware of all these data and definition changes? You cannot. However, you can create an RRT that understands this process. *This gives you the advantage of knowing you do not know*. Not knowing creates a different perspective and can open a "possibilities perspective". One must adopt a logical awareness and balance to incorporate your own strategy for achieving an ability to filter data. Develop and rely on your own judgement—make it a way of living your life. Believe in yourself and trust your intuition. The truth will withstand all scrutiny. Once you have achieved self-awareness you will "sense" a disturbance when data does not seem correct or is incomplete. You will learn to always question the way you filter data. It is OK to be wrong: if you can adapt. Awareness of self allows this to happen. Please remember, you already possess the ability to change; it is just a matter of choice. I cannot stress this often enough. The point here is do you want to change in an aware manner, or an unaware one? This will make more sense to you once you incorporate your quantum awareness processes with the previously discussed pitfalls like Systems of Interference, Lock-on lock-out principle, Reality Replication Templates. Your new awareness understanding is demonstrating how easy it is to become indoctrinated into a way of thinking that creates an invincible and impenetrable shield. Together, we are developing your ability to laugh at yourself and your mistakes so you can just be you. Love the process of learning. Lose all the stress related self-talk. Smile in your never-ending search for information, awareness, self-healing, and consciousness. *Trust yourself to understand LIFE. LIFE continually provides data; learn to identify and use it.*

I have noticed the more aware one becomes to self-healing, the faster you are able to integrate self-supporting awareness (dietary changes, exercise changes, perception changes, etc.) for all areas of your life. A self-healing awareness is pertinent to all the information you accumulate—not just health issues.

Your goal is to connect or, in most cases, re-connect with your innate healing process. This awareness will not only help you with self-healing, but with other *human created detriments*: environmental toxins, semi-effective medicines, disastrous side-effects of medicines, super-strains of diseases, pollutants and more.

Why do we willingly immerse ourselves in toxins and toxic situations? My observation reveals we do so because of complacency, despondency, indifference and in some cases, insanity. Why is so little done to change this situation? For instance, I hear comments like, "I know my car pollutes the environment, but I can't get away from it sometimes. I must drive my car to get to work, school and other places. And yes, I know I am driving in automobile emissions (breathing in those toxins), but there is no other way for me to get around." Ask for help, brainstorm. Minimize or eliminate this exposure and figure out a way to use filters, or even move to a cleaner environment. It is not an all or nothing scenario. Modify the RRT that is making you perceive a negative outcome by being "trapped". Al Einstein once said, "A person with a negative attitude will always bring a problem to the solution.". Anybody can be a "devil's advocate" and tear down possibility thinking. Stay clear of these folks. Surround yourself with people that sculpt the sandcastle, not the ones who kick them down. Concentrate on a positive result—like an inexpensive electric car with filters. The human species has created an un-healthy environment; we are the only ones who can change this.

What is your perception of water (H_2O)? People drink bottled water to avoid the toxins identified in most tap water (a modern reality). However, most of these same people <u>are willing to bathe in the tap water</u> they are not willing to drink! As if tap water, and the toxins it contains, cannot enter your body through your pores. This is not sustainable. Some people tell me it is "un-fair". I cannot afford to have a whole house water filtration system. I simply agree and remind them that your evolution and your survival does not factor in to, "It's un-fair." Toxins, environmental pollutants, and improperly regulated foods affect everyone regardless of race, creed, color, or economic status. *Let us brainstorm and create the impossible.* NOTE: Just because you drink water from a bottle does not insure its clean! When was the last time you had your bottled water tested? Never, once, always? Remember the adage, "Let the buyer beware." The economic factor plays an enticing and significant role in this process and it overrides reason. Be careful.

What causes a species to become extinct? According to The World Counts [8], "The top causes of current extinctions are over-hunting, destruction of habitat, and pollution…destruction of habitats is currently the biggest cause of extinctions." However, all three of these atrocities are caused by humans and therefore can be corrected by humans. Decisive action must be implemented. But when? Only awareness and intention can stop this. **"100,725 species have become extinct <u>SO FAR THIS YEAR – 2019"</u>** says The World Counts publication. [8] "One of Humanity's greatest challenges is preventing the collapse of our food chain." According to the article posted by The World Counts, "Extinctions can disrupt our ecological processes like pollination and seed distribution and cause a collapse of the food chain which can cause more extinctions." [8]

If you state "only the wealthy can eat healthy" you are mostly correct. Isn't the observation that those without money cannot afford clean and nutritious food obvious in many cases? The "heads-up" lesson here is: Figure out a way to include yourself in a quantum survival equation. Let us be the example for others to copy. Collapse this quantum possibility into your reality. Then teach others to collapse the same reality.

Brainstorm with as many people as possible that will listen. (I am helping you right now as you read this chapter with this *awareness. Yep, one of the reasons for this book.*) For instance, why can't your church, synagogue, temple, etc. buy a water filtration system the congregation can utilize before or after you attend their sermons? Could high schools, universities, and other organizations create aquaponics systems to feed students or the community? Wouldn't this help some groups? Let us make these organizations *aware* and turn these gathering places into a **community affair** 7 days a week. Sounds like a win-win scenario to me.

To better analyze and adapt your individual specific situation you will have to be more pro-active for *yourself.* Develop a plan of action which will help support a healthy mind and body (then share it with me and others). I will help pass it along.

The current state of medical awareness is out of balance; no one will deny this. Do not wait for them. You must evolve or get left behind. I know this sounds harsh. Remember, and I cannot say this enough, toxins, medicines, extremely low frequency power emissions, tainted water, etc., do not care who or what you are. They are indiscriminate, mostly man-made intrusive manifestations that *thrive on un-awareness*. These intrusions are the result of the unconsciousness and unaware thinking of our society (yes, we created it). Please, remember it is not about fair; it is about adaptation to the circumstances you are presented with. *Awareness creates possibility.* It is about creating a balanced reality, then showing others how to do the same! You must become involved and ask for help in developing a system which will allow you to move forward and stay healthy. Can a group of people, a school, a university, etc., gather money to build an Aquaponics system to grow clean, nutritious food? Always! The lessons in this book will help you realize possibility thinking. I want you to become a healthy, aware, and self-healing version of yourself--"intend" this to happen. You change the whole world—by changing yourself.

Tragically, medicine has evolved into a capitalistic endeavor to generate money—not health. This aspect must eventually be removed from the equation, but for now, it is the driving force and primary focus of medicine. Employing integral medicine can bridge many aspects of the different medical modalities, but ultimately *you* are responsible for initiating and adapting a strategy that will work for you. How can we, as people, create a viable and sustainable health care system? It will require us to do the impossible—something that survival has done many times before.

The first thing you must "intend" is to augment and support your own awareness of self-healing. Without your intention to do this, it cannot happen. You will be required to become an expert on you. Do not worry, this will become second nature. It must. You cannot dedicate all your time to this endeavor_(unless you are a medical researcher). Your passion should be funneled into your career or life choice, regardless of what that is, Dancer,

Singer, Poet, Lawyer, Engineer, Carpenter, Writer, Computer Tech, Artist, etc. Healing awareness supports your ability to embrace your life's path. Without health, your life's endeavor is incomplete, limited, and short-lived.

The questionnaire below is not designed to make sure you do not get sick. It is designed for self-awareness. It is important to emphasize that *not being sick is not the same as being healthy*. Increase your health awareness to support your innate self-healing process. Create more love in your life, create more laughter, develop aware and intelligent disease prevention techniques, create *individual specific dietary* supplementation—this natural and wonderful conclusion is attainable by any and all who "intend" this.

Questions to Adapt, Evolve and Survive

Integrate the answers to the following list of questions into your self-awareness:

- Do you breathe unclean air; sometimes, all the time, never? How do you adapt for this?
- Do you drink "purified" clean water and then bathe in the same water you will not drink? (Do you think this water does not enter your body through your pores?)
- Do you go to work sick? Sneeze? Cough? Or are you in an area where someone else with a "good work ethic" does this? What is your strategy to

mitigate and deal with this? (Be compassionate and creative to resolve this problem within your workplace.)

- How effective is your immune system? How do you know?
- When was the last time you looked at your entire body with a magnifying glass? I mean this literally. Use a digital photo; front and back (360 degrees). Take a digital photo that you can enlarge to see minute details. Note your observations on paper or a ledger/chart.
- Does your brain work effectively? Any head trauma EVER? How do you know you are operating at your ideal capacity? If not, what is your strategy for repair? SPECT Scan?
- How safe is your home? Are there any electromagnetic fields interfering with your living equation? Are there any powerlines nearby? Etc. What are you doing about it?
- How do you prefer to process data in your environment? Are you aware of Neuro-Linguistic Programming (NLP)? Do you process information as "right-brained" "left-brained" or Kinesthetic? Why is this important to you and others?
- Are you aware of quantum medicine and how it affects your body, mind, and spirit? Are you aware there are other integral medicine options? (See Chapter 13)

- How much electricity is produced when your heart pumps?
- What types of fields does your body use and create? Which dampen your existing field(s)? EMF, electricity, solar, gravity, x-rays, sound waves, etc.
- If you have been diagnosed with (insert your diagnosis here), have you looked at **every major country in the world** to find the best research (track record for researching, treating, and curing this presentation)? Have you looked at examples of miracle cures, spontaneous remissions, placebo effects? These will provide *real life examples of hope* to those willing to make a quantum leap of health awareness and create a support structure for themselves. Which countries are ranked in the top 5?
- Have you looked at Traditional Chinese Medicine and other medical modalities recommended by the CDC and WHO? Why does the CDC and WHO advocate and support Traditional Chinese Medicine if Western Medicine is the preferred modality? Fragments of truth?
- How does your mind store information in your brain? What is Neurogenesis? What is Photonic Encoding?
- How many senses do you use? (19+) Or do you still believe there are only (5)?

- What is a quantum leap of understanding and awareness? How is this used in health and healing?
- How do you determine if you are ailing? According to Dr. Drouin, from Quantum University, Health, Alarm, Adaptation, Exhaustion, Functional, Organic, Death are the seven (7ea) stages of health. How many stages do you use? Most people say I am either sick or not sick. Why not use a more accurate metric and self-aware system description? This description will teach you to become once again more "aware" of your entire self, both physical and non-physical. It also works with any medical modality.
- How many bodies do you have? According to Dr. Amit Goswami, a Physical, Vital, Mental, Supra-mental, Quantum body or God awareness exists. Or are you of the mind set you just have one, your physical body?
- Where am I going with this is more <u>information is better than less?</u> Earlier diagnosis of a detrimental health condition is better than learning about it when it is in its last stages. When would you like to learn you contracted a disease? When it is in Stage #1 or Stage #4?
- How many x-rays have you had in your life? How many X-rays in a one-year period are toxic? How many could cause death?

- Pharmaceuticals: Do you know all the options for treating you? What is the length of time you can consume a prescription according to your pharmacist? What are the side effects? Has the credo, "do no harm" been replaced with "the lesser of two evils"? Write these down.
- Are synthetic compounds easier or harder to assimilate by your body? Why? (Hint: Yes and No)
- Are you unique? Are you different? Do you think you react the same or differently to medicine than everyone else? What can your DNA tell you about this? Should you have a DNA analysis?
- Does medicine affect women differently than men? Which sex (male or female) was used in the drug trials? Why? What about the sex that was left out? How come?
- Why am I asking these questions? What do you think? How do you think?
- Is there another option? (Almost ALWAYS!)
- Is your body temperature the same all day?
- What is your eyesight? Why? How long has it been this way? What caused it?
- When was the last time you had a sonogram, sphect-scan, MRI, f_xMRI, Thermal scan?

- Do you think it is a good idea to learn about yourself now? Or should you wait until you are seriously ill?
- Do you believe your body can heal itself if given an environment conducive of health? Why? What is needed for this to happen?
- New procedures and technology are being developed daily. Name two that pertain to you.

Adapt

To be an aware person, one needs to know their own body and adapt the credo: ***"Do no harm to yourself"*** Become knowledgeable about every aspect of yourself. No one can put more time into this objective than you. Nor can anyone know "your" awareness of your body—this *must* be done by you and it must include both the physical and non-physical aspects of yourself. Learn to become your own primary medical information provider. You will need to collect on-going data to help produce the best evaluation of who you are at any given time. If you come up with a spectacular way of organizing and collecting this data share it with others; as this collection process will always be evolving. I believe any good doctor or practitioner ALWAYS wants as much information as they can get (regardless of the medical modality) about your presentation. When it comes to understanding your specific presentation of symptoms during your visit to their office for treatment, more is better. More information about what makes you tick, makes the differential diagnoses process much more definitive and accurate. If your doctors and other medical professionals are not interested in the data you have collected, ask them why. Better yet, find a doctor that wants this information. Your practitioner needs to establish trust and a sense of overall caring for "you". (This goes both ways.) Find a doctor who will review your collection of objective and subjective data. Hopefully, they will suggest you track other observations about yourself that you can add to your list. Some of the data you collect will be physical data like measurements for height and weight. Other data can be photos, notes about various colors on your body and other skin observations including your tongue, graphs of your blood pressed and pulse, and much more. Look into the latest technology to help collect this data.

Some of the data you collect will be an extrapolation of data which is non-physical: cognitive, psycho-social interpretations, logical extrapolation of non-local data (like how you feel, what emotions your experiencing, etc.). It is also important to note how much time you spend in front of a computer, physical activities. **Learn what makes you, YOU.**

Evolve

Does the Flu care who or what you are? When a flu strain is identified, search the entire globe to understand its presentation and analyze cures. Does the ingestion of Mercury only affect the poor? The obvious conclusion is "No". To evolve is more than just not being sick. It is not just a DNA change, it's a combination of epigenetic data and Photon Information Expressions combined with your DNA which can make you a stronger version of the human species; it's about fulfillment of your life's passion in a manner that allows more love, happiness, laughter, singing, dancing and yahoo! It is about re-connecting to the awareness of all living organisms.

When LIFE expressions are in balance, as a species, we will experience an awareness that will eradicate previous unconsciousness—a quantum leap. It is important to remind you that this book is not about you changing the world. This book is about the awareness of you changing you. The noticeable collateral effect is a healthier and more balanced awareness of our world—this is your quantum gift to this collective reality.

Chapter 16

"If we were to examine our diseases poetically, we might find a wealth of imagery that could speak to the way we live our lives." –Thomas Moore

Quantum Awareness and Plants

Plants are essential in supporting your body's immune system. This support of phyto-healing (plant healing) properties appears to be more "balanced" and easier to assimilate into your body when an entire plant compound is used, as opposed to a single constituent. This can include leaves, bark, roots, etc. Reductionistic science identifies specific constituents in plants as the "active ingredients" that eliminate or mitigate a specifically observed malady. These ingredients do things like reduce fever, or they are anti-biotic or anti-fungal. The isolated constituent is then used as a medical treatment option. This approach is not always the best option. The observation is:

(1) The purpose of removing this constituent from a plant implies the other constituents present in the compound are not necessary, only the individual specific constituent. NOTE: It has been my experience with patients that the whole medicinal plant exhibits phenomenal energetic and bio-chemical synergistic qualities. Why are all the other constituents present in a compound? Do they create balance within the living compound? Aren't plants chemists too? Why does a plant include the other constituents?

(2) An isolated constituent is patentable; the entire natural compound is not.

(3) Many synthetic Medicinals can cause side effects if they are not IDENTICAL to the constituents copied from nature. [1]

The human species evolved and sustained life for thousands of years as hunter-gathers. Humans either ate plants and fungi or ate animals that ate plants and fungi. For the most part, those were the only options. For thousands of years the human physiology adapted and evolved predicated on this survival diet strategy. Today's humans eat synthetic food substances. Not all synthetics are bad if produced *identical* to their counterparts grown in nature. However, trusting "those" that have a financial interest to provide a pure product can prove challenging. Humans eat pharmaceuticals, they breathe unclean air, they drink unclean water and are subjected to environmental toxins (poisons) which are life threatening. Additionally, most of the humans I have met are *addicted to sugar*. I believe it is difficult for the human body to digest most synthetics substances, including the almost identical versions of synthetic substances due to the absence of the other naturally occurring constituents grown by nature. It is self-evident that the bodies of humans and other species have a difficult time adjusting to synthetic and toxic substance intrusions. Ask yourself what the "side-effects" are of the synthetic substances you are ingesting? They are not hiding. You are the one hiding from the answer. When your body rejects *anything* there must be a reason. Trust that your body normally provides your best analysis and response—a continuous self-healing and maintenance response. Hiring a chemist and medical research scientist is a good idea to become aware of how and why.

At this point in human history, a strong self-awareness is mandatory. Always monitor your own body. Know your body and mind. This will give you the advantage of having current and accurate data to provide to your doctor or the medical professionals you choose to help you.

Humans consume synthetic, unnatural substances and secrete them into our environment via sewage treatment facilities and it has been shown to have a detrimental effect on the environment. (100's of tons a year; it is sad this is now common knowledge.) This has already caused the extinction of many organisms. [2] If these substances are killing the environment, what makes you believe this is not affecting your physical body and the billions and billions of micro-organisms that live inside you? How many parts per thousand, per million, or per billion can you ingest before experiencing negative effects? Have you ever thought about how small parts per thousand, per million or per billion are? Once again, this information is not hidden. When was the last time you checked to ensure this data was current and correct? Who makes this determination? Why is it legislated? This *awareness* alone should give you cause for immediate concern—and concern for our environment. Investigation can reveal the truth. This must be done by you so you can experience this firsthand.

Thankfully, “live” plants help. When used properly, plants and other micro-organisms can mitigate and eliminate many environmental toxins (Yeah!). Plants existed on earth many millennia before humans. [2] Many animals existed before humans. [3] Many of these plants and animals have collapsed waves of possibility into reality without the use of humans which is evidenced by their material reality and examples of their quantum reality expression. In other words, you can see they exist. Being “conscious” is NOT exclusively a human awareness. It is a quantum field awareness. Consciousness is observed in other plants and animals. (See Chapters 10 and 11 on Plant Intelligence and the Bumble Bee orchid.) Humans are dependent on plants for food, clothing, and medicine. *Plants are vital to our existence—a quantum survival equation.* As you develop self-healing awareness you will learn to work in harmony with plants, and your environment. Reconnect with their beauty, their intelligence, and their predominately peaceful existence.

As previously discussed, the mechanism for collapsing quantum possibilities into particles of reality are photonic interpretations constructed in your mind, a non-local information awareness field. But, not necessarily or exclusively the human mind, as evidenced with the bumble bee orchid and other plants and animals. The experience humans refer to as” life” integrates all quantum collapses occurring in one species. These choices are used toward the fulfillment and continuation of those organisms. This data resists entropy and is contained within this universe as Photon Information Expressions, a Live Intelligent Information Field Expression and a Total Information Continuum). Dr. Amit Goswami states, "To collapse a quantum wave of possibility into a particle of reality; one requires observation and conscious thought." [4] This continues until a death-transition is experienced by that organism **(QP + SA + O/M + I = QR)** or quantum possibilities + sapience + observation/measurement + intention = quantum reality.

QP = Quantum Possibilities

SA = Sapience

O/M= Observation/measurement

I= Intent

QR= Quantum Reality.

The bumble bee orchid exhibits intelligent design and awareness (See Chapter 10, Bumble Bee Orchid) as well as non-local cognitive experiences like sentience and sapience. However, any "existence" is observed as non-local and requires a cognitive methodology when extrapolating data to support a definition. The human mind experiences 20,000 to 70,000 [5] of bits of thought data per day. This infers intelligent selectiveness on the part of the *thought experience process* as to what is recorded permanently and what is recorded temporarily or not at all (a Reality Replication Template). **Humans think in photonic expressions, see in photonic expressions and dream in photonic expressions.**

Humans create an image-based reality. I believe this is how the brain and mind record sensory data that is imprinted and or combined with photonic expressions (images). It is logical to extrapolate that we store these data in our physical brain using direction from a non-local construct (LIFE), which utilizes thought expressions from the (mind). This experience uses your own mind's ability to select data and directs the brain to *create a physical manifestation* to store this data in.

The projection screen of the mind, so to speak, or the way the mind views this image-based data, is experienced as an invisible mental construct. This view is perceived in humans as directly in front of our eyes and is especially noticeable when they are closed. This viewing area seems to have a limited scope or field of perception since the photonic images are centered in front of our eyes with no apparent peripheral imaging. Additionally, there are no images above the head or below the chin area of the head. Moving or repositioning the head does not interfere with this perception. This viewing screen construct is observed as an *awareness experience light expressions* (EMS) capable of analyzing and recalling all sensory data from the brain by using *intention* to do so. This non-local viewing screen, so to speak, can also utilize information obtained from its non-local environment which has *not* been recorded in the brain (Like my "sudden knowing" experiences).

Thinking can create new synapses (neurogenesis) [6] or new ways which cause actual physical changes in human brain tissue. These "creations" are new ways of assimilating and processing data. The “thinking” observation **($K^r + P^r = MA$)** literally updates your perception of data using the recording and retrieval aspects of your brain. This allows the mind to be more aware of itself in relation to the data it collects and analyzes. This augmentation of new data is the result of a living organism’s individual specie specific intent to know. From this quantum experience a physical manifestation occurs—a reality perception. All data accumulated by a living organism is modified by its awareness or RRT. This is a logical extrapolation. Why keep or accumulate data if you are not going to use it? This also applies to the awareness perceived from quantum leaps regarding the changing of original (old) data or our new realization (awareness/perception) of that old data. *It should be noted that “awareness” is not predicated on education. Rather, it is the product of introspection, self-analysis, and an intent to know.*

The more frequently sensory data is utilized by a living organism, the more likely it is to create a template of these “repeated experiences” or a Reality Replication Template. It is logical to assert that memory, or recalled data, is always filtered by a subjective perception due to RRTs being individual specific. Therefore, the recalled data is not necessarily an exact copy, but an *approximate or variant copy*. It should also be noted that Systems of Interference are present in this data. SI creates incomplete conclusions that need to be acknowledged and accounted for during this subjective awareness experience.

When new *information* is experienced it takes the place of the old data. This makes the previous data incomplete and obsolete (this is a quantum leap). The resulting change causes your perception and knowledge to be instantaneously changed. This new awareness replaces the interpretation of the previous data.

It is estimated there are 37 - 40 trillion cells in the human body. Additionally, human brain cells continually grow, expire, and transform for repurposing. [7] The conscious mind immediately has the brain create new neuro-synapses and deactivates old synapses [7] that create data changes in human memory. This is your "you specific" reality awareness—a new egoic understanding.

Intent is a non-local mind construct [8] or thought expression experienced by you. Intent directs specific inquiry with a pre-determined target or goal as a desired result. Intent is evident in the thought processes of living organisms and is exhibited as a thought expression or idea.

It is self-evident that science constantly evolves, giving support to new discoveries which supersede previous "factual data". The importance of saying this is not to restate the obvious, but to alert the reader to the trap! Until we discover the new data, *we operate under the assumption that the old data is correct.* This "absolute knowing", LOLO effect, promotes an almost impenetrable "you specific" definition (RRT) and makes it extremely hard to accept new information due to these Systems of Interference. If you "know" or even think you "know" a piece of information is factual, there is a tendency not to question your own perception of your knowledge.

I have observed and believe "thoughts" are photonic images that are non-local data field expressions (See Chapter 5, Photonic Encoding). This photonic data is acted upon by your intent and filtered by a "you specific" analysis. This is your interpretation of the picture, so to speak. As previously discussed, this is evidenced by the ever-present photographic image presentations which are observed with all thought expressions. When you select or recall a thought expression from your brain to be acted upon by your mind, a *representative photonic* image appears. This is how a thought expression is represented to you *regardless of the physical sensory data used to create this thought.* A thought is an expression observed in what appears to be a quantum field (picture screen) as a manifestation experience (a photographic image). We describe and define a "thought expression event" in terms of encoded sensory data—holographic images (as a picture).

Photons = Ph

Thought* = *T

Sensory data = Sd

Intent = I

Systems of Interference = SI

Using *intent* while directing photonic representations stored in the brain, and/or the experiencing of new data plus Systems of Interference, results in a *thought experience* or a thinking analysis. Intent that acts upon photons + sensory data + systems of interference = Thought or **(I ->Ph + Sd + SI = T)**. Intent is non-material. It is a state of mind that refuses to be quantified in a reductionistic science model due to its non-material properties. This can only be defined using a cognitive (qualitative) science model. The word "intent" resists clear definition and becomes ambiguous when alluding to Merriam-Webster's definition, which states, "The state of mind with which an act is done." [9] What does this mean? What is a state of mind? Logic dictates it is not material and that the "intent experience" provides a way to produce a desired result. Our aim, target, or intent in this book is to compile useful definitions and request that antiquated or incomplete definitions be revised. This type of analysis insists you ask questions. As you have seen, definitions can prove difficult at times.

I = Intent

K = Knowledge

P = Perception

MA = Manifestation of Awareness

SI = Systems of Interference

Intent acting on repeated knowledge and perception and mitigated by Systems of Interference creates a manifestation of awareness or **$(I + (K^r \leftrightarrow P^r) + SI = MA)$**. Reason is defined by Merriam-Webster as: "Think, understand, and form judgments by a process of logic."

[10] Sentience + Reason + Memory + Modified Awareness = **Sapience** or **(S + R + Res + MA = SAP)**. Sapience is not predicated on being a human. It is predicated on a definition: **If any LIFE form fulfills the requirements defined for being sapient, then, by definition, they are sapient**. However, this does not infer sapience in all organisms is equal. Varying degrees of sapience exist. Problems associated with the "all or nothing concept" can be systematized to create a guideline for reasonable analyzation.

Is thinking a closed system of review; an analyzation originating from the brain? I believe no. This really does not support the observation. Thinking is a non-material construct. I believe thinking is a quantum field expression event which does not originate in the brain. It is an awareness that exists in a living "information field" which can access the mind. Remember, the mind directs the brain to create places to store thought, a process known as neurogenesis. Additionally, like radio waves, this Live Intelligent Information Field Expression of Photonic Information is transmitted/emitted everywhere as a frequency of the EMS of radiation and is available to anyone or any device that can intercept and receive this type of wave/particle data.

Remote viewing experiments performed by the United States CIA support this assertion. [11] The mind is a non-local quantum field experience. It is self-evident. There are no physical or material components present. I believe the human brain is physical and records all sensory data by super imposing or combining data with photonic images (Photonic encoding). These data expressions are received by a non-local experience referred to as the mind or mental body. The received information is used in conjunction with the physical brain and memories. Intention can be used to affect or direct this retrieval of information. However, as previously mentioned, logically, "anything or anyone" that is tuned to the same frequency can receive it. Afterall, what are humans if not information collectors?

Being willing to experience awareness (using intent) creates a fertile environment for exposure to the Live Intelligent Information Field Expression. Yes, you can change your self-awareness, augment your ability to self-heal, and receive healing information just by utilizing "intent" to do so. Using intent and belief affects self-healing. Some examples of this self-healing effect are exhibited as the placebo effect, spontaneous remission, and miracle cures.

Chapter 17

"The present finding, along with those from conceptually similar experiments, suggests that the disclosure of trauma is simultaneously associated with improvement in certain aspects of immune function and physical health."—Dr. James Pennebaker

"Search with new eyes for the photonic expressions of life."—Dr. G. Munger

The Placebo Effect, Spontaneous Remission, Miracle Cures

Miracle Cures

According to Dr. Robert H. Shmerling of Harvard Medical School, "Research into the pros and cons of the placebo effect has changed how many people think about this phenomenon. We used to think the placebo effect was limited to suggestible people with a "real" disease; we now know better." [1] I believe collapsing quantum waves of possibility into particles of reality with focused intention aimed at an end-result (like a cure), is responsible for the placebo effect. You are literally creating the end-result you want to achieve with LIFE (just the way you create yourself). Isn't this a belief coupled with intention? Couldn't a quantum equation be responsible for this? I believe it is plausible that the implementation of data received from a Live Intelligent Information Field, a quantum expression, is responsible for this phenomenon. Most researchers agree there is nothing physically present in a placebo treatment that can affect a disease or condition. A placebo effect is observed, upon implementation, to be a *belief-thought, a non-local awareness manifestation.* A human can create a "thought" by implementing a quantum intention to do so (you are doing it right now "thinking" about this assertion made by me). As previously discussed, *intention* exhibits an awareness of *your* ability to create a reality expression (you are aware that "intention" can create your desired goal). In the case of a placebo, the effect is a belief in cure, your desired cure! You do this type of creating every day when making your own Reality Replication Template. Remember, you create you. I believe this same quantum equation is responsible for self-healing and healing-awareness—an awareness that includes the placebo effect.

There are countless examples of placebos which are self-evident, so you will have no trouble looking up multiple examples on the internet.

The progression of our discussion of self-healing and self-awareness is leading you toward direct examination of evidence, the preferred methodology for investigating self-healing (be careful of ambiguous definitions and "everybody knows" assumptions). What do you observe when you or a patient directly experience a placebo effect? Do you feel better and experience changes? What do you believe this non-local phenomenon is? It is obvious this must be a non-material "something" which is influencing, mitigating, or curing the disease. What else could this be? Is it logical to conclude a Live

Intelligent Information Field Expression might be responsible? Let us investigate.

I believe the existence of this morphogenetic-like field expression exhibits life and intelligence and is an organized field expression. There are too many *live* variables to contend with that can and do change for this field not to be alive. An intelligence expression of some form would need to be present to interpret and integrate these variables of data, so to speak.

I believe our quantum human awareness is co-creating humanity's next step toward creating a brain (neurogenesis) with expanded abilities. This new brain would be able to receive and comprehend new data frequencies—data which will change life and reality as we know it (this observation is progressive; it/and you, are already doing it!). Think about this and remember to include ALL your observations while utilizing both quantitative and qualitative methodologies (a system integration approach) as you analyze any data.

Hold onto your hat, here we go!

Spontaneous Remission

This brings us to the phenomena of spontaneous remission (SR) of a disease or cancer. No scientist will state these phenomena do not exist. They are definable and observed as actual case histories, but they elude quantification (using a stand-alone quantitative methodology)—we do not know the mechanism that allows these phenomena to occur (yet!). Maybe it is time to investigate quantum fields that record and transfer all data, LIFE.

Caryle Hirshberg and Brendan O'Regan define spontaneous remission as "the disappearance, complete or incomplete, of a disease or cancer without medical treatment or with treatment that is considered inadequate to produce the resulting disappearance of disease symptoms or tumor."

Remember, multiple thousands of SR cases have been documented. [2] [3]

How can we use a quantum medical awareness understanding and a self-healing awareness to predispose us to experience these phenomena? First, you have to decide whether the thousands of documented spontaneous remission cases (and growing!) fit in your Reality Replication Template. Do you believe this data is pertinent to your current presentation? Ask your doctors, show them the data. Remember, as mentioned above, as of the date of this writing, thousands, and thousands of cases of different types of cancer presentations at different stages of development have experienced spontaneous remission, not just a lucky few. Wouldn't this be worth looking in to? Your choice.

The above observations meet the requirements for the definition of hope: Spontaneous remission *exists,* so the *hope* to experience spontaneous remission as a cure is valid. Additionally, when you state there is "no hope of a cure", given the thousands upon thousands of examples of spontaneous remission, you offer false hope. Do not worry, your chosen doctor will help you sift through the data and examples (these case histories are online, you can bring these examples with you for a joint analysis).

However, ultimately this is an individual specific decision made by you and your doctor. Logically, you would read everything you possibly can about your specific presentation of disease. You would counsel with EVERY medical professional that will listen to you. You will evaluate their expertise and weigh the pros and cons of the data you received from: Medical doctors, Nutritionists, Naturopathic doctors, Ayurvedic doctors, Tibetan doctors, Oncologists, Herbalists, spiritualists and more. Search the entire planet for data related to *your* diagnosis and *your* prognosis, not just the United States. You will also want to speak with the spontaneous remission survivors who have the same diagnosis you now have—the more the better (this also provides a support group to whom you can ask questions and share intimate or frightening concerns). These doctors, health professionals and survivors experiencing spontaneous remission will help provide you with information to make an informed decision on how *you* want to proceed with your treatment.

Kelly A. Turner, PhD, wrote a book, *Radical Remission.* [4] Dr. Turner offers compelling examples of spontaneous remission (SR) and correlates data from her own research from around the world which offers nine key factors associated with SR survivors. There are many books to choose from, (Lisa Rankin wrote, *Mind over Medicine*. Institute of Noetic Sciences published *Spontaneous Remission: An Annotated Bibliography*, by Caryle Hirshberg and Brendan O'Regan). The point here is they all have one thing in common—*there exists multiple ways to successfully treat disease*. Reviewing case specific SR data bases and case histories is a logical approach.

Normally, fear and anxiety are associated with any life threating diagnosis. This is where your awareness training comes into play. Remember, get to know the body and mind aspects of your individual specific health presentation (What makes you, you). This will augment the discovery portion of your learning process (knowledge of self) and expand the understanding associated with your perception of this knowledge **($P^r + K^r = MA$)** and self-healing awareness.

Some doctors have "theorized" that spontaneous remission is just part of the disease's natural progression. However, I have yet to see any logic which supports this assertion. You cannot state spontaneous remission is just a natural progression of a disease and that you will uncover the actual process of how it works at a future date. That does not tell us anything. A theory must be based on logical extrapolation of existing empirical evidence or observation of a visible result, not a future speculation.

The following cases of spontaneous remission are just a sampling of the kind of data that is starting to become common place and is being accumulated by researchers all over the world. The NOEITC.ORG library, listed below, published a 713-page report [3] on spontaneous remission in 1993; imagine how much larger it is today!

From *Immunity over inability: The spontaneous regression of cancer* Thomas Jessy states, "In our relentless efforts to go beyond nature to fight cancer, we often overlook the facts nature provides to heal our maladies." Another quote from the same abstract is, "It is interesting to note that the current primary cancer management procedures neither harness the benefits of patients' own immune system nor stimulate it to achieve tumor regression **but actively suppress it; thus it does not run parallel to [the]body's own defensive mechanisms, but opposes its natural role**." (Emphasis mine) This is the third and last quote, and one I hope will intrigue you to read these observations, "…while acute infection, fever, and cancer vaccines by the virtue of immunostimulation induce regression of cancer even in the most advanced stage of disease and prove that cancer is **not** an irreversible process without a cure." [5] (Emphasis mine)

Fever, cancer incidence and spontaneous remissions authored by: Kleef R, Jonas WB, Knogler W and Stenziger W. and published with PUBMED state the following conclusion: *"Pyrogenic substances and the more recent use of whole-body hyperthermia to mimic the physiologic response to fever have successfully been administered in palliative and curative treatment protocols for metastatic cancer.* **Further research in this area is warranted."** [6] (Emphasis mine)

Another published example is:
Spontaneous regression: a hidden treasure buried in time by Hoption Cann SA[1], van Netten JP, van Netten C and Glover DW. The following is from their Abstract: "Spontaneous tumor regression is a phenomenon that has been observed for hundreds, if not thousands of years. Although the term spontaneous implies 'without apparent cause', a review of case reports over the last several hundred years demonstrates that regression generally coincides with acute infections. Observations of this non-specific effect led to the emergence of active cancer immunotherapies by the 1700s. By the 1890s, William Coley refined this approach with a bacterial vaccine which, when administered properly, could induce complete regression of extensive metastatic disease. Unfortunately, after Coley's death, his vaccine and technique fell into obscurity. Modern approaches to treatment have reduced the occurrence of spontaneous regressions. Aseptic techniques and antibiotics significantly reduce postoperative infections, while chemotherapy and radiation impair immune activation even when an infection does occur. More than a century after its inception, Coley's vaccine and aggressive approach to treatment may still be one of most effective immunotherapies for cancer." [7]

Another important study is *The Toxins of William B. Coley and the Treatment of Bone and Soft-Tissue Sarcomas* by Edward F. McCarthy, MD. The following is from the Abstract of this study: "In 1891, William B. Coley injected streptococcal organisms into a patient with inoperable cancer. He thought that the infection he produced would have the side effect of shrinking the malignant tumor. He was successful, and this was one of the first examples of immunotherapy. Over the next forty years, as head of the Bone Tumor Service at Memorial Hospital in New York, Coley injected more than 1000 cancer patients with bacteria or bacterial products. These products became known as Coley's Toxins. He and other doctors who used them reported excellent results, especially in bone and soft-tissue sarcomas.

Despite his reported good results, Coley's Toxins came under a great deal of criticism because many doctors did not believe his results. This criticism, along with the development of radiation therapy and chemotherapy, caused Coley's Toxins to gradually disappear from use. However, the modern science of immunology has shown that Coley's principles were correct and that some cancers are sensitive to an enhanced immune system. Because research is very active in this field, William B. Coley, a bone sarcoma surgeon, deserves the title "Father of Immunotherapy"

Each year in the United States approximately 5000 people die from bone and soft-tissue sarcomas.[1, 2] These deaths occur despite innovative techniques in surgery, new chemotherapeutic drugs, and the sophisticated delivery of radiotherapy. Therefore, to reduce this death rate, new treatment modalities are being investigated. One such treatment modality is immunotherapy.

Immunotherapy is based on the idea that a patient's immune system can be stimulated or enhanced to attack the malignant tumors (Emphasis mine). The first systematic study of immunotherapy for the treatment of malignant tumors was begun in 1891 by William B. Coley (1862-1936), a bone sarcoma surgeon (Figure 1). Coley injected streptococcal organisms into a cancer patient to cause erysipelas and stimulate the immune system. The patient's tumor disappeared, presumably because it was attacked by the immune system. This experiment began Coley's life-long study of immunotherapy. For the next 40 years, he treated hundreds of patients with inoperable bone and soft-tissue sarcomas using immunotherapy. His work was widely publicized and discussed. He was in the ideal location to carry out his work as the Chief of the Bone Sarcoma Unit at Memorial Hospital in New York, America's first cancer hospital, and his work was supported by the first cancer research grant, which he helped establish." [8]

It is evident from the evidence presented above, that more research is warranted in this area. It is also evident that *all* medical modalities need to exert a concerted effort to expand and catalog spontaneous remission of disease examples in a database that anyone can access for **free**.

I believe the Photon Information Expressions in a human body influence the quantum signature known as "you". As we have been discussing, you can collapse quantum waves of possibility into particles of reality. You are the co-creator of your existence and the most influential contributor to your Reality Replication Template. In addition to this, you are the custodian of your physical body. As you are learning, you can help this process or impede it, your choice.

Miracle Cures

The list of miracle cures is a loooong list! Many miracle cures have been attributed to religious experiences from 196 countries, 4,200 religions, and 80,000 variations of these religious beliefs by 7.7 billion humans on our planet. (Whew!)

These religious healings exist in various forms from deity intervention to the belief constructs attributed to individual specific religious interpretations, to everyday individuals' interpretations (quantum belief expressions). Trying to do a competent meta-analysis of these accounts would be an endeavor that spanned several lifetimes. However, one observation is common in all these miracle cure examples: *It is a belief (a quantum thought analysis) which is predicated on a subjective understanding that promotes a desired end-result—resulting in a cure).* The point I am stressing is this a "belief construct" (a quantum thought expression) not a material substance which is being administered to an ailing person to cause a healing effect. This "belief construct" is something else; it is not material. I believe this "belief construct" is quantum data. It is this information which provides the orchestration to the material body to affect a cure.

This common observation is a non-local experience which mitigates or eliminates a disease or malady in a physical body and oftentimes imbalances mental states (psychological imbalances). This infers a live, intelligent, organized quantum field expression. After all, what is a "belief" if it is not a subjective belief of a quantum expression? Additionally, as we have already discussed, an actual quantum belief expression does not conform to humanity's predominately material evidence-based interpretation of medicine. This would account for those who choose to interpret a different type of healing reality, like SR. The empirical observation of "how is this done" does not affect the end-result. In other words, if a miracle cure, placebo effect, or spontaneous remission occurs as an example of a healing awareness, embrace it until the day when we can quantify "how this is done". We do not know how this happens—but it is documented to happen!

Al Einstein said, "The most beautiful and profound emotion we can experience is the sensation of the mystical. It is at the root of all true science. That deeply emotional conviction of the presence of a superior reasoning power which is revealed in the incomprehensible universe, is my idea of God." I agree. **Search with new eyes for the photonic expressions of life.** And please, help others to see this aspect of themselves.

Chapter 18

"...Physical reactions are observed and exhibited in a material body due to experiencing an emotional event."—Dr. G. Munger

Mind-Body Interactions Are Self-Healing

When an emotional event (happy, sad, glad, angry, etc.) presents as a "perception experience", a "thought expression" occurs in your mind. This "thought expression" is predicated on information retrieved from your non-local environment and incorporates one or more of your senses (sight, hearing, smelling, etc.) from your material environment. This results in **P < - > K = A**; or perception affects your knowledge and knowledge affects your perception (a feed-back loop). These are combined to create awareness.

An interesting phenomenon occurs when this happens. *Physical reactions are observed and exhibited in a material body due to experiencing an emotional event.* For instance, if you receive information that ***you*** consider "sad" you might experience some of the following physical reactions:

1. crying and tearing
2. abnormal breathing, panting, groaning
3. physical retraction/contortion
4. blood pressure change
5. mucous flowing from your nasal membranes

6. frowning
7. pain

If you received information *you* considered "happy" you might experience some of these physical reactions:

1. crying
2. abnormal breathing
3. blood pressure change
4. smiling
5. physical contortions associated with laughter

These two examples exhibit physical changes occurring in a material body that are predicated on "perception-events". These physical changes were caused by a "thought expression" or a series of "thought expressions" which were non-material. This means these "thoughts" are non-local expressions. This conclusion states quantum expressions (thoughts) apply an observable physical effect directly to a "live" material expression and directs or orchestrates these physical reactions. This orchestration requires the "quantum expressions" to be intelligent, organized, and able to interact with the quantum aspects of the material body. I believe these Photon Information Expressions must be alive and intelligent to react and interact due to the incomprehensible variables observed which mitigate the unpredictable and ever-changing events present in a live organism (See Chapter 7 Live Intelligent Information Field Expressions—LIFE).

What is the purpose of these physical reactions? Do these physical reactions help restore a material body back to its state of equilibrium or homeostasis? *The observation is a qualified yes; meaning it is dependent on the varying degrees of awareness which are mitigated by your Reality Replication Template—your belief filter.* Nevertheless, let us examine why some of these physical reactions occur:

Crying can be described as tears (a saline rich solution) being secreted from the eyes which are part of the material body. I believe the human body is "aware" of these secretions (See Chapter 6 Live Intelligent Information Field Expressions). These observations are easily seen and felt and create an awareness experience. I believe the presence of Photon Information Expressions directs the continued construction and maintenance of this material body. Why tears? Are tears removing something detrimental to the physical body? Is there something being removed that is causing an overload? It sure looks that way. Are tears carrying "information expressions of emotional overload" out of the physical body? What is your baseline observation for the constituents in your tears? What is your observation for tears secreted during sadness? Are these specimens the same? What is your observation for tears of joy? What are the results of a spectrographic analysis or gas chromatography analysis of your tears, prior to and post?

Tears can be the way the material body reacts to an emotional overload. *Is the physical body removing this quantum thought expression via your tear ducts?* Should we test "tears" to see what type of crystalline structure it exhibits? Dr. Emoto's studies on water show "field expressions" are carried by water (Tears are mostly water!). As you can see, we could write a scientific paper exclusively on "tears". This research paper is "crying out" to be completed by Doc Emoto (more humor). The point of this example is "self-awareness" and awareness of the self-healing mechanisms involve quantum fields. Probably, no one has pointed this out to you before; now you know.

What about breathing? Does the "human body" benefit from short breaths, long breaths, intermittent breaths, panting, etc.? There are copious amounts of research on the benefits of breathing regimens. Why does *the body choose* and exhibit the observed breathing changes during emotional experiences? Does this seem to be an intelligent, organized, self-healing response? What is regulated by a breathing response? Field imbalances? Cardiovascular presentations?

This bring us to blood pressure fluctuation. The heart is an intelligent organized sub-system (organ or specific grouping of cells) of the human body akin to the brain. Why does the heart change your blood pressure to increase or decrease—an observed cardiovascular response during an emotional event? Do *you* think this cardiovascular response is a self-healing response? I sure do. Why does this response slow or speed up your hearth rate? It appears to be an intelligent and organized response to a quantum field expression (an emotion). Can emotions affect your heart and cardiovascular system? I say yes, what do you think?

Why is smiling or frowning present during most emotional events? Why do muscles, tendons, skin, and tissue move in specific directions in response to smiling? Why only these muscles, tendons, and specific types of skin? What is happening during this process? Do these physical reactions create blood flow to specific areas of the body? How does this promote homeostasis? Does a smile or frown communicate emotional qualities to the environment (photonic images)? What do you think the purpose of a smile is? A frown?

Lastly, what are the reasons the human body contracts or contorts during pain, laughter, crying, etc.? Do these physical movements increase the flow of blood, lymph, etc., to the areas of the body experiencing movement, like laughing and jumping or contorting? Do these physical movements decrease (or increase) the flow of blood or lymph to the areas of the body experiencing the movement, like when your body is contracted in a fetal position? How does this affect endorphins?

Aren't all the above observations self-healing, self-awareness, self-adjustment? Aren't all these physical responses intelligent, organized and individual specific to the organism and their Reality Replication Template? Being aware of these observations allows you to augment and understand their beneficial effect for your body. As previously discussed, becoming aware is accomplished by utilizing intent to do so.

Some healing responses are: Crying, abnormal breathing, panting, groaning, physical retraction/contortion blood pressure change, mucous flowing from your nasal membranes, frowning, pain, sleeping, cellular regeneration, sneezing, coughing, burping, vomiting, scratching, fever, sleep, fasting, yawning, physical movement, etc. and intentions or RRTs (good or bad, these are combined with your ignorance or awareness which support this process).

The following is an end of chapter question: What is the purpose of "turning red" or blood rushing to your face when you are embarrassed? Mind/body reactions can be examples of self-healing. Self-healing and self-awareness contribute to an understanding of ourselves and to how we as a species interact. We can choose to help by choosing to become aware.

Chapter 19

"Never doubt that a small group of thoughtful, committed citizens can change the world. Indeed, it is the only thing that ever has." –Margaret Mead

How Can All of Us Help?

A natural part of health-awareness is sharing self-healing experiences. This is important, since the mutually shared connection of a "malady experience" has the potential to create deep understanding and emotional support, a support that promotes healing using real-time examples. When you share your individual specific self-healing experience, it creates an opportunity for others to relate to your experience (You are forming a Group Reality Replication Template). This is profoundly important. The emotional impact of being diagnosed with certain diseases and cancers can be overwhelming to most people. I believe having a support group is warmly welcomed. It is my wish to provide support by presenting "healing possibilities".

Humans and other organisms collapse quantum waves of possibility into a material reality by the mere act of observing and intending "their" reality to exist. What a gift! This is truly a magical reality expression—meaning a currently unknown scientific or spiritual explanation of how this is accomplished. However, I believe it exists as a live, organized, quantum field expression.

The data bases listed in Chapter 18 are a spectacular resource for those of us that wish to study some of the effects of self-healing. These case histories and anecdotal examples of "other than" thinking, demand analyzation. These examples should be continuously studied and disseminated to all who wish to examine *known examples* of self-healing. In addition to these multiple data bases which house the above mentioned spontaneous remission examples, other examples (yours!) should be included. If you, or anyone you know, has experienced spontaneous remission, you should add your story and ask others to add their story to the growing list of examples being reported from all around the world. The goal here is to create a global data base. This will allow researchers to collect evidence and endeavor to observe any similarities in this group that could facilitate a better understanding or intuitively point research in a direction for a cure.

This must be a group effort aimed at collecting data on spontaneous remission for the purpose of identifying the commonalities which have been identified. These "commonalities' lead the thinking mind in the direction of discovery. Reviewing these case histories, like the list Dr. Kelly A. Turner, PhD is amassing [1] creates support for those afflicted and provides more data to facilitate *possibility* thinking. We, as a group, must be willing to exhibit universal care, compassion, and cohesion toward the collection of data which has the potential to further awareness and research, and more importantly, save lives.

Chapter 20

"Nothing is impossible, the word itself says I'm possible!"—Audrey Hepburn

Conclusion

The focus of this book has been to explore new revelations and bridge old understandings and insights. Self-healing and self-awareness will foster an evolved understanding of your life. Our investigation has provided you a way to discover your individual specific signature—*you.* You have learned the value of continually observing the aspect of yourself that presents as a Reality Replication Template. You have discovered that everyone and all other life forms collect information from their environment differently. This is an individual species-specific endeavor. This process has created a self-evident new awareness in you. You have discovered you can understand this innate process. A process that was already a part of "you". It just needed to be pointed out to you again. You have learned how to use "intention", a quantum thought expression of focused desire to produce real, observable change. You learned to observe LIFE from a different perspective. A perspective I believe embraces Photon Information Expressions (PIEs)as *alive, aware, and intelligent.* This is the observation of the "living animation effect" you observe when looking at yourself and others. These "field expressions" are extensions of a universal live intelligent force field or an intelligent

Live Information Field Expression (LIFE). This original LIFE is a group of infinite field expressions that utilize PIEs to transmit and receive data to and from all "life equations" living on our planet. This book posed the question: Why can't there be *alive* "fields" that are not based on human interpretation? These fields are quantum observations. After all, **life existed before humans**. Humans appear to resist any evidence or observation that demote them to an intelligent mammal, part of a quantum continuum—part of a field expression. This human GRRT is a blind spot in this awareness and reeks of anthropomorphic bias and diploma mill indoctrination. We have learned that science and spiritual philosophies are striving to understand the same enigma—LIFE.

Science does not impede spiritual conviction. Science reaches out for enlightenment—the same is true for those who seek spiritual enlightenment. The blending of these two approaches has always been apparent. Afterall, spirit is non-material. It is a "quantum expression" *described* the same in all religions as non-local or non-material. The Systems of Interference humans created has caused this separateness. I hope this book created a bridge, even if it is only the first stone that embraces investigational methodologies as both independent and interdependent on each other. Our goal is one and the same—a quest to know. With intention and love, we have the power to create signs on **both sides** of this bridge which read, "**Welcome**".

We established the observation that self-healing is experienced in varying degrees by everyone. Our discussion of how to utilize and augment self-healing invites us to consider concepts and new understandings that provide the *opportunity for change*. You learned new awareness concepts that are mandatory in your understanding of how you create you. Concepts like how you record sensory data from your environment (photonic encoding), definitions and how they affect your reality, "things" that interfere with your egoic interpretation of life (Systems of Interference, LOLO effect and RRTs), and the importance of knowing *your* mind and body intimately. You now can finally become who you have always been. Attaining this awareness is your gift to yourself and the world. This awareness is embodied in your Reality Replication Template(s) and change is predicated on your willingness to "intend" something different.

An augmented self-healing awareness is available to you just for the asking. Please remember, *you are essential in your own cure. All healing is self-healing and is predicated on a live information field that provides healing data and your intent to use this awareness*.

With love and great expectation,

George

Gratitude

Thank you for our shining star
A glowing globe of fire
It warms our skin, our life, our soul
A sight you can admire
We must include Mother Earth
A host to you and me
Her skin provides a place to live
And everything we need
Please remember all the plants
That live with us and sway and dance
A festival of life's romance
For everyone to see
Recall the gift of water
Imbued with life itself
Loved by all creation
A liquid form of health
I introduce awareness
Of love and friends with smiles
An Infinity of connectedness
That makes our lives worthwhile
Eternal love Ex^{2}pressions

From perfect living hosts
For without their loving synergy
We would just be ghosts
Dr. G. Munger

Glossary

Throughout the course of this book several new equations and new or expanded definitions were used to help clarify the material being presented. The following glossary defines these equations and definitions in a manner that clarifies their purpose and usefulness. NOTE: Some are defined by outside sources and the quoted source is listed.

Aware is defined by Merriam-Webster [6] dictionary as “having or showing realization, perception or knowledge.”

Awareness is defined as knowing or detection.

Cognitive Science is defined by Merriam-Webster dictionary as “an interdisciplinary science that draws on many fields (such as psychology, artificial intelligence, linguistics and philosophy) in developing theories about human perception, thinking and learning. [7]

Electromagnetic Spectrum is defined as all the frequencies and/or waves in the known range of the electromagnetic spectrum radiation.

Emotion is defined by Merriam-Webster [8] dictionary as “the affective aspect of consciousness. A state of feeling.”

Field Expression is defined as a collective in which each individual part is comprised and affected by a unifying force resulting in a single or combined group presentation.

Genome is defined as all the DNA and genes in a complete living organism.

Holographic Images is defined as light images and encoded data.

Instinct is defined by Merriam-Webster [9] dictionary as "a natural or inherent aptitude, impulse or capacity – a largely inheritable and unalterable tendency of an organism to make a complex and specific response to the environmental stimuli without involving reason – a behavior that is mediated by reactions below the conscious level."

Intelligence is defined by Merriam-Webster [10] dictionary as "the ability to learn or understand or to deal with new or trying situations – the ability to apply knowledge to manipulate one's environment or to think abstractly as measured by objective criteria." (such as tests)

Intent is defined by Merriam-Webster [11] dictionary as "the state of mind with which an act is done – a usually clearly formulated or planned intention – aim."

Intention is defined as thoughtful purpose.

Knowledge is defined by Merriam-Webster [12] dictionary as "the fact or condition of knowing something with familiarity gained through experience or association – the fact or condition of being aware of something."

Photon Information Expression (PIE) is defined as a living, intelligent, organized, group of photonic expressions which collect and transfer data to a Total Information Continuum, which is part of a live intelligent, interactive, information field—an entity expression."

Live Intelligent Information Field Expression (LIFE) is defined as a universal, live, intelligent, organized, self-aware field comprised of seemingly infinite photonic information expressions. It can also be referred to as a quantum continuum or spiritually, as God.

Local is defined here as an observation directly associated with material surroundings.

Memory is defined by Merriam-Webster [13] dictionary as "the power or process of reproducing or recalling what has been learned and retained especially through associative mechanisms – the store of things learned and retained from an organism's activity or experience as evidence by modification of structure or behavior or by recall and recognition."

Non-local is associated with non-material expressions and observations.

Perception is defined by Merriam-Webster [14] dictionary as "a result of perceiving – observation – a mental image –concept – awareness of the elements of environment through physical sensation color perception – physical sensation – physical sensation interpreted in the light of experience – quick, acute and intuitive cognition – appreciation –a capacity for comprehension."

Photonic Encoding (PE) can be described as a process in which the mind and physical brain of humans or a neural-like-network (NLN) in other organisms coordinate the recording and retrieval of environmental sensory data to and from the brain or NLN, as photonic images (holograms) and not the actual sensory data input experienced.

Phyto-sapience is defined as a plant's ability to be aware of and consciously interact with its environment and exhibits the ability to think, reason, and demonstrates the capacity for memory of data which can be recalled later (Coined by me).

Phyto-sentience is defined as a plant's ability to be aware of and consciously interact with its environment (Coined by me).

Plant Intelligence is defined as a plant's varying degree of sapience that exhibits an awareness of their environment, themselves, the ability to think and reason as well as the capacity for data memory that can be recalled at a later time (Coined by me).

Quantum Phyto-Sapience is defined as the ability of a phyto-sapient plant to observe and select quantum waves of possibility and collapse them into particles of reality (Coined by me).

Reality is defined by Merriam-Webster [15] dictionary as "the quality or state of being real – something that is neither derivative nor dependent but exists necessarily in reality – in actual fact."

Reason is defined by Merriam-Webster [16] dictionary as "a statement offered in explanation or justification – the power of comprehending, inferring, or thinking, especially in orderly rational ways – intelligence."

Sagacious is defined by Merriam-Webster [17] dictionary as "of keen and farsighted penetration and judgment – discerning like a sagacious judge of character – caused by or indicating acute discernment."

Sapient is defined by Merriam-Webster [18] dictionary as "possessing or expressing great sagacity."

Self-awareness is defined as detection or the ability to be cognizant of a thought which is happening to you, both physically and mentally (local and non-local).

Sentient is defined by Merriam-Webster [19] dictionary as "responsive to or conscious of sense impressions."

Spirit is defined by Merriam-Webster [20] dictionary as "an animating or vital principle held to give life to physical organisms – soul – temper of disposition of mind or outlook, especially when vigorous or animated – in high spirits – the immaterial intelligent or sentient part of a person – the feeling, quality or disposition characterizing something undertaken."

Systems of Interference (SI) is defined as preconceived ideas which mitigate/manipulate information in a manner so that it superimposes unrelated data for inclusion or exclusion in an equation, experiment or reasoning process. This includes economic bias, predetermined outcome of an experiment, anthropomorphic bias, racial bias, religious bias, social mores, political bias, group/mob mentality, gender bias, diploma mill indoctrination, or any other blind inclusion or exclusion of unrelated data. (Coined by me)

Think is defined by Merriam-Webster [21] dictionary as "to form or have in the mind – to have as an intention – to have as an opinion – to regard as – consider –to reflect on – ponder – to call to mind – remember – to devise by thinking – to form a mental picture of."

Thought is defined by Merriam-Webster [22] dictionary as "an individual act or product of thinking – a developed intention or plan – the action or process of thinking – cogitation – serious consideration – regard – reasoning power – the power to imagine – conception."

Understanding is defined by Merriam-Webster [23] dictionary as "a mental grasp – comprehension – the power of comprehending – the capacity to apprehend general relations of particulars."

EQUATIONS

Quantitative Process

(D+Q+ROR = Proof of hypothesis) However, in some examples when quantification cannot be ascertained we can use: **(D+ROR=Proof** when the result exists in a material form.

Definition of Problem= (D)

Quantification= (Q)

Replication of Results= (ROR)

To clarify the cognitive scientific model's observations, I proposed the following equations—delineated below. According to Dr. Amit Goswami, "the individual-specific reality (conditioning) or egocentric reality, is what most live organisms, including humans, experience due to their inability to filter out their subjective interpretation. All observed and recalled data are subject to this individual's specific interpretation or perception." [1]

Knowledge (K), affects Perception (P) and P affects K; this is an example of a circular concept or feed-back loop **(K <-> P is circular ∞)** which can produce new change and create new awareness in one's own individual specific database of knowledge and perception. This new awareness is collected from the environment by using your senses. This process allows new and old thoughts to be experienced repetitively. This happens regardless of where the knowledge is stored. The data can be re-collected from the brain as memory or experienced as new environmental sensory data in the mind in conjunction with the brain. An exchange of data is observed in both the conscious and sub-conscious mind. This can be logically deduced because all individual human memory is stored data which exists in a single physical brain. [2] Consequently, memory is accessible in both a conscious state and an unconscious state or dream state as evidenced while sleeping. Currently, this circular exchange of data is observed to be limited by the life span of the organism (If a human body lives to be 100 years old or 3,153,600,000 seconds, then this is your individual specific time frame to compile data to and retrieve data from your brain). To accomplish this, you must use your mind and the quantum expression of intent. It is important to note the physical mechanism used for storing data (the brain) denigrates and transitions (recycles) at some undetermined point in the flow of time. This makes infinite possibilities using this process (the brain) impossible due to the death-transition of the material form.

Ergo, if perception changes knowledge and knowledge changes perception, then **(K + P = A)** is a representation of awareness. However, this is only theoretical. This is due to the fact that if perception and knowledge are continually repeated$^{(r)}$ it creates a modified awareness or **(P <-> K then, $K^{(r)}$ <-> $P^{(r)}$ = MA)**. This equation is important because it sets up the preferred mental environment and opportunity for augmenting one's ability to experience an instantaneous change in awareness that irrevocably replaces past conclusions and beliefs (a quantum leap). This modified awareness is the form all humans utilize to interpret their environment and is individual specific. [3]

P + K = A (only theoretical)

P -> K and K -> P a feedback loop or circular concept

P <-> K ∞

($K^r + P^r$ = MA)

(P <-> K then, $K^{(r)}$ <-> $P^{(r)}$ = MA)

Knowledge affects Perspective

Perspective affects Knowledge

Knowledge = K

Knowledge repeated = K^r

K <-> P is circular ∞

Perception = P

Perception repeated = P^r

Awareness =A

Modified awareness =MA

Modified awareness repeated = MA^r

Reality Replication Template = RRT

<u>Modified awareness repeated = (MA^r = RRT)</u>

(Sd + MA = S) = Sentience

Modified Awareness = MA

Sensory Data = Sd

Sentience = S

Sensory data combined with modified awareness is observed to be a form of Sentience.

(rSd + MA + Res = SA)

Sensory Data = Sd

Sentience = S

Sapience = SA

Reason = Res

Modified Awareness = MA

Memory or recalled sensory data = rSd

Recalled sensory data (memory) can affect change of your perception in a modified awareness model. Additionally, when this equation is expanded to include reason it fulfills the requirements of sapience [4] "or the quality of the state of being real" (which is included here for ease of continuity).

QP = Quantum Possibility

rSd = Memory (retrieved data from the brain)

R = Reality

Res = Reason

SR = Subjective Reality

SI = Systems of interference

S = Sentience

SA = Sapience

O = Observation

QR = Quantum reality

PSA = Phyto-sapience

PE = Photonic Encoding

I = Intent

(A +QP + rSd + SI + SA = SR) = Subjective Reality

(QP + SA + O + I = QR) = Quantum Reality

(QP + PSA + O + I = QPS) = Quantum Phyto-Sapience

These observations require me to account for how sensory data is received, stored, and recalled by the human brain. I believe Photonic Encoding is the system utilized by the mind and brain to make these interpretations (See Chapter 5, Photonic Encoding). Wikipedia states [5] , "In quantum mechanics, wave function collapse is said to occur when a wave function—initially in a superposition of several eigenstates appears to reduce to a single eigenstate (by observation)."

Ergo, to collapse a wave function, one needs to observe a quantum wave of possibility and experience a sense an individual specific expectation that confers intent to collapse the quantum possibility into a particle of reality.

SA = Sapience

O = Observation

I = Intent

QP = Quantum Possibility

QR = Quantum Reality

QPS = Quantum Phyto Sapience

This equation states: Quantum possibility + Sapience + Observation + Intent = a particle of reality or **(QP + SA + O + I = QR)** a quantum reality. An example of plant sapience is the bumble bee orchid. Its version of this equation is essentially the same: Quantum possibility + Phyto-Sapience + Observation + a feeling of conscious intent = a particle of reality or

(QP + PSA + O + I = QPS) or Quantum Phyto-Sapience.

References

Preface

[1] https://www.ncbi.nlm.nih.gov/pmc/articles/PMC3052954/

Chapter 1: How do YOU become YOU?

[1] https://libguides.usc.edu/writingguide/quantitative

[2] https://www.livescience.com/21456-empirical-evidence-a-definition.html

[3] https://www.amazon.com/Radical-Remission-Surviving-Cancer-Against/dp/0062268740

[4] https://libguides.usc.edu/writingguide/qualitative

[5] https://www.techopedia.com/definition/9614/system-integration-si

[6] https://www.quora.com/What-is-the-difference-in-lay-mans-terms-between-Newtonian-physics-and-quantum-physics/answer/Nikolas-Scholz

[7] Goswami, A. (2008). *Creative Evolution* (First Quest Edition). Theosophical Publishing House, P. O. box 270, Wheaton, IL 60189-0270: Theosophical Publishing House.

[8] https://www.sheldrake.org/research/morphic-resonance/introduction

[9] Goswami, A. *Physics of the Soul*, p 123,

[10] Brockman, John. *This Idea is Brilliant* (2018), p 401

[11] Campbell, S. (2011). The lock-on/lock-out principle, p 11

Chapter 2: Self-Healing

[1] https://www.merriam-webster.com/dictionary/heal

[2] https://www.merriam-webster.com/dictionary/curing

[3]

https://www.researchgate.net/publication/232074348_Herbert_Frohlich_FRS_1905-1991_-_A_physicist_ahead_of_his_time

[4] https://www.brainpickings.org/2012/02/21/brian-cox-everything-is-connected/

Chapter 3: How YOU Affect Everything

NONE

Chapter 4: A New Perspective

[1] https://www.dictionary.com/browse/quantum--leap

[2] https://biblehub.com/john/8-32.htm

Chapter 5: Photonic Encoding: New Revelations on How the Mind and Brain Work

[1] https://en.wikipedia.org/wiki/Sensory_processing
[2]

https://www.google.com/search?rlz=1C1CHBF_enUS877US877&sxsrf=ACYBGNQfkdZXr0XvW2kPltaaalnj0NnHuw:1576275689748&q=free+image+of+the+electromagnetic+spectrum&tbm=isch&source=univ&sa=X&ved=2ahUKEwj9urjE1LPmAhVVrZ4KHV64CzkQ7Al6BAgIECQ&biw=1536&bih=722&dpr=1.25

[3]

https://www.bing.com/search?q=electromagnetic%20radiation%20spectrum%20of%20visable%20light&qs=n&form=QBRE&sp=-1&pq=electromagnetic%20radiation%20spectrum%20of%20visable%20light&sc=2-51&sk=&cvid=A3CF5DF3FA4D4F6094809BF321EF1004
[4] https://en.wikipedia.org/wiki/Sound
[5] https://en.wikipedia.org/wiki/Sound
[6] https://www.merriam-webster.com/dictionary/sound?src=search-dict-box

Chapter 6: Auras and Emanations are Photonic Expressions

[1]

https://www.bing.com/images/search?q=Bioluminescent+Plants&FORM=IRBPRS&=0
[2] https://www.theguardian.com/science/blog/2009/jul/17/human-

bioluminescence
[3] Humans Glow in the Dark, para. 2,

https://www.theguardian.com/science/blog/2009/jul/17/human-bioluminescence

Chapter 7: Live Intelligent Information Field Expressions

[1] https://en.wikipedia.org/wiki/LIFE
[2] https://lms.iquim.org/course/view.php?id=235

[3] https://www.dictionary.com/browse/LIFE
[4] https://www.merriam-webster.com/dictionary/alive
[5] www.thegaurdian.com/science/blog/2009/jul/17/human-bioluminescence

[6] https://www.cia.gov/library/readingroom/docs/CIA-RDP96-00789R003300210001-2.pdf

[7] https://www.bing.com/images/search?q=Real+Near-Death+Experiences&FORM=RESTAB
[8] people.eku.edu/ritchisong/birdnests.html

Chapter 8: Problems with Definitions

[1] https://www.merriam-webster.com/dictionary/definition

[2] https://pixabay.com/illustrations/atom-science-research-physics-1013638/

[3] https://nationalpost.com/news/world/stunning-image-of-a-single-strontium-atom

[4] https://www.merriam-webster.com/dictionary/kill

[5] https://en.wikipedia.org/wiki/List_of_carnivorous_plants

[6] https://en.wikipedia.org/wiki/LIFE

Chapter 9: Live Plants Support Self-Healing?

[1] https://www.merriam-webster.com/dictionary/intelligence
[2]

https://www3.rps205.com/programs/PublishingImages/Pages/Renaissance-Testing- /CogAT%20Information.pdf

[3] https://islandpress.org/books/brilliant-green
[4] https://www.scientificamerican.com/article/plants-attract-enemys-ene/
[5] https://www.scientificamerican.com/article/plants-attract-enemys-ene/

[6] https://www.scientificamerican.com/article/plants-attract-enemys-ene/
[7] philosoplant.lareviewofbooks.org/?p=96
[8] https://www.southerndestinations.com/incredible-acacia-tree-phenomenon/

[9] https://io9.gizmodo.com/10-pieces-of-evidence-that-plants-are-smarter-than-you-5901172
[10] https://www.plantsci.cam.ac.uk/news/2013-10-23
[11] https://en.wikipedia.org/wiki/Intelligence
[12]

https://www.sciencedaily.com/releases/2007/10/071004143133.htm
[13] www.indefenseofplants.com/blog/2016/4/17/the-sexual-ruse-of-the-bee-orchids
[14] https://www.youtube.com/watch?v=-lwYj_GwGiQ
[15] Orchids imitate insects that pollinator fights.
https://www.bing.com/images/search?q=orchids+inmate+insects+that+pollinators+fight&go=Search&qs=ds&form=QBIR
[16] ttps://www.youtube.com/watch?v=Y9dhcEW9-7c

Chapter 10: The Bumble Bee Orchid (Ophrys-Bombyliflora

[1] Trewavas, A.
https://en.wikipedia.org/wiki/Ophrys_bombyliflora
[2] Cvrckova, Lipovsha, & Zarsky 2009,
www.ncbi.nlm.nib.gov/pmc/articles/PMC2676749

[3] Bohman, B., Phillips, R. D., Menz, M. H., Berntson, B. W., Flematti, G. R., Barrow, R. A., Peakall, R. (2014). Discovery of pyrazines as pollinator sex pheromones and orchid semiochemicals: Implications of the evolution of sexual deception.

Retrieved from PubMed:
www.ncbi.nlm.nih.gov/pubmed/24697806

[4] Pheromones and animal behavior., Retrieved from: users.ox.ac.uk/~abrg/pheromones/documents/Wyatt-introtopheromones2hs.pdf
[5] Deceptive flowers orchids., Page 1, Para. 5., Retrieved from: blogs.britannica.com/2011/03/deceptive-flowers-orchids/
[6] Munger, G. PhD, Quantum Phyto-Sapience Chapter 12 of this book

Chapter 11: Sentience and Sapience of Plants

NONE

Chapter 12: How to Support Self-Healing

[1] Merriam-Webster def of sentient

[2] Merriam-Webster def of sagacity

[3] Merriam-Webster def of sentience

[4] Numerous studies on plant intelligence

[5] Goswami's quote: "In quantum physics, objects are depicted as a possibility (a possibility wave) yet when an observer observes these possibilities, they collapse into an actuality (the wave collapses into a particle)"

[6] Stephen Hawing: "A researcher's intent can skew the results of an experiment"

Chapter 13: Types of Medical Modalities

[1] https://quoteinvestigator.com/2017/10/23/be-change/

Chapter 14: Subjective Memory Experiment

NONE

Chapter 15: Analyze, Adapt and Evolve

[1]

https://www.google.com/search?source=hp&ei=tX1hXf7BEYCS0

PEPl5ikwAU&q=definition+of+LIFE&oq=definition+of+LIFE&gs_l=psy-ab.3..0i70i249j0l9.1056.8461..11909...0.0..0.142.2018.1j17......0....1..gws-wiz.......0i131j35i39i70i249j35i39.oaWe9hbHHIE&ved=0ahUKEwi-8J3DjZzkAhUACTQIHRcMCVgQ4dUDCAc&uact=5

[2] Drouin, P. (2015). Creative integrative healthcare training, Seven stages of illness. Retrieved from: https://lms.iquim.org/course/view.php?id=235

[3] Wikipedia. Definition *of* alive

[4] https://www.merriam-webster.com/dictionary/alive?src=search-dict-box

[5] Kobayashi, M., Kikuchi, D., & Ohamura, H. (2009). Imagery of ultra-weak spontaneous photon emission from human body are displaying diurnal rhythm. Retrieved from PloS One: www.ncbi.nlm.nih.gov/pmc/articles/PMC2707605/

[6] https://www.cia.gov/library/readingroom/document/cia-rdp96-00787r000500250015-6

[7] https://www.theatlantic.com/magazine/archive/2015/04/the-science-of-near-death-experiences/386231/

[8] www.theworldcounts.com/stories/Causes-of-Extinction-of-Species

Chapter 16: Quantum Awareness

[1] https://novarecoverycenter.com/drugs/synthetic-drugs/ [2] https://www.theguardian.com/science/blog/2014/aug/08/drugs-toilet-pharmaceutical-pollution

[3] Marshall, Feb. 1, 2012, para. 4

[4] Wikipedia, March 14, 2018, p. 1

[5] Goswami, A. (2008). *Creative Evolution* (First Quest Edition). Theosophical Publishing House, P. O. box 270, Wheaton, IL 60189-0270: Theosophical Publishing House.

[6] http://blogs.discovermagazine.com/neuroskeptic/2012/05/09/the-70000-thoughts-per-day-myth/

[7] Berlang, C. (Feb. 06, 2017). How do neuroplasticity and neurogenesis rewire your brain? Retrieved from: www.psychologytodya.com/blog/the-athletes-way/201702/how-to-do-neuroplasticity-and-neurogenesis-rewire-your-brain

[8] https://www.collective-evolution.com/2016/02/07/physicists-examine-consciousness-conclude-the-universe-is-spiritual-immaterial-mental/
[9] https://www.merriam-webster.com/dictionary/intent
[10] https://www.merriam-webster.com/dictionary/reason
[11] https://www.cia.gov/library/readingroom/docs/CIA-RDP96-00789R003300210001-2.pdf

Chapter 17: Placebo Effect, Spontaneous Remission and Miracle Cures

[1] https://www.health.harvard.edu/blog/the-placebo-effect-amazing-and-real-201511028544

[2] http://www.ncbi.nlm.nih.gov/pmc/articles/PMC1888599

[3] https://library.noetic.org/library/publication-bibliographies/spontaneous-remission

[4] Turner, Kelly A., PhD a book, *Radical Remission*: Surviving cancer against all odds. (2014), Harper Collins Publishers, first edition, ISBN 978-0-06-226875-4

[5] https://www.ncbi.nlm.nih.gov/pmc/articles/PMC3312698/

[6] https://www.ncbi.nlm.nih.gov/pubmed/11549887/

[7] https://www.ncbi.nlm.nih.gov/pubmed/11812185/

[8 **Chapter 18: Mind-Body Interactions are Self-Healing**

[1] https://www.ncbi.nlm.nih.gov/pmc/articles/PMC1888599/

Chapter 19: How Can We Help?

NONE

Chapter 20: Conclusion

NONE

Glossary

[1] https://www.merriam-webster.com/dictionary/definition

[2] Drouin, P. (2015). Creative integrative healthcare training, Seven stages of illness. Retrieved from: https://lms.iquim.org/course/view.php?id=235

[3] https://www.merriam-webster.com/dictionary/kill

[4] http://www.sarracenia.com/faq/faq1120.html.

[5] https://en.wikipedia.org/wiki/LIFE

INDEX

K

L

M

N

P

Q

R

S

Y

www.ingramcontent.com/pod-product-compliance
Lightning Source LLC
LaVergne TN
LVHW021745071126
851857LV00039B/742
* 9 7 8 0 5 7 8 2 2 9 6 9 0 *